RAPID WEIGHT LOSS HYPNOSIS FOR WOMEN

RAPID WEIGHT LOSS HYPNOSIS FOR WOMEN

STOP EMOTIONAL EATING PROVEN STEPS AND STRATEGIES FOR LOSING WEIGHT REPROGRAMMING YOUR SUBCONSCIOUS MIND BY USING SELF HYPNOSIS

Kyleigh Wyatt

Kyleigh Wyatt

Contents

1

Introduction

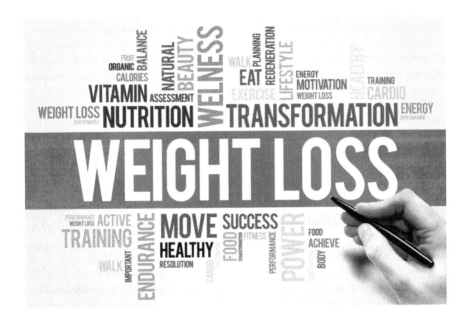

Losing weight is something almost everyone wants to do. It seems so easy to quit a specific type of food or to do exercise or to follow a specific food and exercise pattern for a week. But it takes a lot of determination and motivation to carry on this process.

Hypnosis is among the new methods that are being used to help overweight people lose some pounds. Several ways come under the umbrella of hypnosis, but detailed visualization is one of the primary methods used for weight loss.

Hypnosis seeks to establish an extreme degree of patient focus while inducing positivism into the unconscious mind of the person. It also helps cultivate a sense of well-being inside the individual and makes him more confident about the whole weight loss process.

Many people are confused as to how exactly hypnosis will help them with weight loss.

Hypnosis by itself is not a weight-loss treatment but instead a means by which you can adhere to your regimen.

You will be reeducating the unconscious mind by hypnosis to think positively. You are going to be more confident and able to stick with your plan.

Hypnosis explicitly aims to reach into one's mind and change their way of thinking. While this seems obvious, you do need a weight loss solution, and if your mind forgets about it afterward, then you may have difficulty finding ways to achieve your goals.

This book contains proven steps and strategies for reprogramming your subconscious mind by using self-hypnosis and unleashing the hidden power within which you have been longing.

Take the time to study and follow the given instructions. You will find that upon completion of this, you will not only have the ability to change virtually any area of your life for the better, but you'll also be able to do the same for the lives of your family, friends, and loved ones.

I know that this guide would help you put your best foot forward.

This might not be a fix-it-all guide, but it sure sets the correct tone. Now it's time to go out there and put your best effort into the test. Be the person you were meant to be.

Hypnosis for weight loss is basically using hypnosis techniques to allow you to lose weight. It is a way to shed a few extra pounds. But most of the time, it is paired with a diet plan.

You should continue with a good dietary regimen, followed by a moderate exercise routine. This will allow you to lose weight faster, and if you are a person who has cravings, then this will also help you immensely.

You will be able to get help on your issues regarding food, and this form of hypnosis will allow you to have a better time with your cravings. You can do this with a professional, but you can also do it on your own. It will let you have control of your life, and, therefore, those bad cravings you have.

While reading this, chances are you are also in a very relaxed and suggestible state. So, whatever is said here should be taken literally but not so much so that it overwhelms you. You will use mental images to convey the meaning of the words that are spoken. You will have your attention focused on that, and when your mind is in a state of concentration, you will start to have your subconscious handle your cravings.

With hypnosis for weight loss, you will allow yourself to view your body in a positive way. It's a great way to take life by the horns.

By doing this, you'll be able to control the factors in your life, such as stress or how much you eat, and turn them around when necessary to give yourself a more positive image that will benefit you in ways you've never expected before.

You will be guided on how you can achieve the maximum benefits of hypnosis and hypnotherapy for weight loss.

So, without further ado, let's turn the page and learn the secrets of hypnosis.

2

Food Addiction

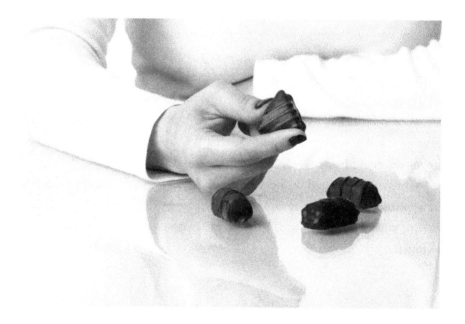

Dealing with Food Addiction

How does a food addict's brain differ from a naturally lean brain? This section describes the most characteristic differences within the mind, especially in food addicts:

- We are crazy about food.
- We usually force us to eat.
- We need more food to be full.
- We often suffer from hunger.

- We respond more strongly to food references.
- Emotional imbalance causes brain hunger in us.

Functional Magnetic Resonance Imaging (fMRI) uses the magnetic properties of blood to work out which area of the brain is most active when it experiences a specific event. Neuroscientists can measure brain activity when food addicts are exposed to food labels, or eat certain foods.

"It's like training," explains Dr. Ashley Gerhardt. "When you train a specific muscle, blood flows into that area.

The brain seems to be working in a similar way, and you'll track which area of the brain receives blood first."

The fMRI consistently shows that the convergence zone for sensory information is that the prefrontal cortex, associated with reward stimuli, particularly primary reinforcement factors like food. To elucidate the neurobiological mechanisms by which weight, mood, and age affect the appetite response, Dr. Gerhardt presented some photographs of foods with different fat content and caloric density to healthy, average weight, and obese adolescent and adult women while undergoing fMRI (high reward vs. low reward). She showed that food-addicted women view highly rewarding foods the same way drug addicts view drugs.

Dr. Bart Hoebel, originally from Princeton University, was among the primary team that tested mice for sugar addiction. He showed that each drop of sugar they swallowed increased the amount of dopamine.

Almost like human addicts, Hoebel's sugar-rat developed a hypersensitive dopamine receptor that was hyperresponsive to specific medicine, and its changes were long-lasting. Even after a month of self-discipline, the taste of sugar would cause the rat to become addicted once again.

In a similar study in Birmingham at the University of Alabama, Dr. Mary Boggiano found out that a food attack in rats elicits an equivalent pleasing receptor within the brain that drug addicts stimulate once they ingest drugs. Dr. Boggiano's oleo-conjugated rats had long-term changes in endogenous opioids within the brain and became abnormally receptive to delicious food.

The dopamine reward system makes us feel good and is related to obsessive gambling, drug abuse, and sex. Food satisfaction results from several similar neural signals and pathways that also regulate orgasm. As a result, many neuroscientists have begun to record that obesity, eating disorders, and even healthy appetite resemble addiction. "Repeating dopamine over and over is what drug abuse does," says Dr. Hoebel. "This causes you to wonder if food may have addictive properties."

"Food gives you a distinct physiological response the same way that drug consumption gives you an enormous response," says psychiatrist Walter H. Kaye, director of the Eating Disorders Program at the University of California, San Diego.

The drug takes over the food reward. "Drugs are addictive because they open the way for appetite."

Like other drug therapies, food therapy is an effort to release the dopamine levels required by all addicts.

During a 1954 study with pleasure centers, two McGill University researchers, Dr. James Olds and Dr. Peter Milner, documented the consequences of dopamine.

During this study, rats had the option of pushing a bar to electrically stimulate the pleasure center or push another bar for food. Dr. Olds and Dr. Milner said the electrical stimulation of rats towards the pleasure center was more rewarding than eating. The experience was so satisfying that the hungry rat ignored the food for the pleasure the electrical impulse from the pleasure center gave it. Some rats stimulated the brain more than 2,000 times per hour for twenty-four consecutive hours. Most rats died on an empty stomach.

Heroin and cocaine addicts also happen to quit eating and lose tons of weight while taking the drug. This fact explains why you get dopamine fixes from other sources. That is also the primary stage of affection, with all the activities that we find so enjoyable, we forget to eat or don't eat that much! The poison is high dopamine, not food.

If this mechanism fails, we find ourselves eating an excessive amount of food, hooked into repairing the lost dopamine.

So, that's why you overeat. You do not eat because you wish it, but because you're compelled to consume.

Types of Overeating

Based on the above rationale, the habit of overeating is often divided into two types:

OBSESSIVE OVEREATING

Dr. Gearhardt, a scholarship recipient at the Yale University Rudd Center for Food Policy and Obesity Center, conducted a neurobiological study and documented similarities in how the brain responds to drugs and delicious foods. Like drug addicts, food addicts struggle with increasing appetite and are encouraged to check their triggers to food and retain control when consuming excessive quantities. Even as one drink can send a recovering alcoholic on a bender, biscuits can trigger an obsessive overeater.

"The results of this study back the idea that increasing expectations for food may partially cause forced diets," said Gearhardt.

Counting on the expected food intake, participants with higher levels of food obsession showed more activity within the parts of the brain alleged to create the motivation and urge to eat than with suppression of inhibiting mechanisms during impulses.

Gene Jack Wang, MD, director of drugs at the Brookhaven National Laboratory in Upton, NY, and Dr. Nora Volkow, director of the National Institute on substance abuse, had this perspective on human imaging studies and grilled chicken. The smell of hamburgers and pizza releases dopamine into the brain. This food stimulus significantly increases dopamine levels within the minds of gluttons, but not in non-gluttons. The quantity released correlates with the intensity of one's desire for food for an extended time, and so the subjective impression is to go and "look for it."

"This is how our brain controls our desires," said Dr. Wang. Many food addicts feel weak in their ability to regulate when and how much they eat. The brain unit contains the striatum, a neighborhood of the emotional brain that contributes to motivation, and therefore the neurotransmitter dopamine, which controls the search for pleasure and produces pleasure. "Now we're not just talking about balancing the energy state," he says. "We are discussing human psychology," said Wang.

COMPULSIVE OVEREATING

The ventral striatum of the brain is best known for its role in motor pathway planning and coordination. Still, it's also involved during other cognitive processes, including executive functions like memory. In humans, the striatum is activated by reward-related stimuli, but also by aversive, novel, unexpected, or intense triggers; and, therefore, the symptoms related to such events. If you see the brain like a train, the striatum on the ventral side is the accelerator.

When food enters the body, it stimulates the pleasure center, which increases the flow of dopamine. When overeating becomes standard behavior, three things happen:

- The reward system is kidnapped,
- Neuroplastic changes occur,
- Serotonin and GABA (inhibitor) neurotransmitters involved within the "brake system" are reduced.

Food addiction confuses pleasure centers. It's more like when the brakes of a train break down, and runaway trains eventually get off the tracks. They are all accelerators, no brakes. Forced or compulsive overeating is like this.

Why Do We Overeat?

Eating is one of our biological needs and is ensured by the enjoyment we feel once we do it. But as soon as we get hooked on food, like long-term alcoholics become ready to drink everyone under the table, and as drug addicts need more and more medicine, we develop a higher tolerance to food. All kinds of addiction require increasingly more addictive substances to raise dopamine levels. Chronically strong drinkers have few signs of addiction, with high blood alcohol levels, which are either impossible or fatal to non-drinkers.

Tolerance facilitates the consumption of overconsumption of alcohol, which results in future physical addiction. Similarly, the addict's brain needs more food to supply the amounts of dopamine that are related to normal high-grade foods.

Men who consume a lot of web pornography are a great example of this type of phenomenon. The men that completely rely on this type of dopamine fixation report that they're unable to be happy or satisfied during intercourse with a real woman. They might go months without visiting an X-rated website and endure severe withdrawal symptoms before they finally regain the enjoyment of interacting with a real woman.

In 2001, alongside his colleagues, Dr. Volkow, including Dr. Wang, obtained brain scans of overweight and normal-weight volunteers to review the enumeration of dopamine receptors. Dr. Wang noticed that overweight people had fewer dopamine receptors; the more obese they were, the less of these important receptors they had. He says the brains of overweight people and drug addicts are strikingly similar: "Both have fewer dopamine receptors than normal subjects."

All addicts are trying to find an answer, but if we become more immune to our drugs—in our case, eating food—a little amount of non-delicious food reduces the feeling of joy and results in the underproduction of dopamine. Something stagnates within the process of the generation of dopamine within the brain.

Genetic damage is named polymorphism. If one among the genes required for the dopamine process may be a polymorphed, it'll appear in certain people with prominent symptoms.

Again, dopamine is a neurotransmitter produced by our brain when we enjoy something. Once you enjoy a delicious salad, vegetables, or slice of pizza, you might want to roll in the hay because your mind produces a healthy amount of dopamine. So, overeating is forcing us to repair dopamine.

The misconception that fat women have more fun while eating than thin women is flawed. The fMRI again shows that a healthy brain produces far more dopamine than the mind of a food poisoner. Food addiction has an equivalent adverse effect as other addictions. The addicts develop a greater tolerance for their drugs of choice, and low dopamine levels mean less experience of pleasure. Therefore, most addicts consume a large amount of food once they want to release the expected amount of dopamine. This fact is one of the apparent and measurable differences between a naturally lean female brain and an obese female brain.

This phenomenon explains why we act absurdly if we don't reach the food levels that cause the assembly of dopamine that is enough to experience pleasure.

Food poisoners suffer overwhelming of hunger within the presence of food. Overeating obsessively and compulsively when not hungry means they are more vulnerable to smells and a strong desire to eat, even after a full meal. Researchers call this phenomenon "external food hypersensitivity." British Medical Research Centre presented a study during which brain scans have shown how this food susceptibility affects people's diets.

When we are hooked into overeating, our brains are programmed to use food to temporarily relieve anxiety, frustration, stress, depression, agitation, and discomfort with dopamine modification. The longer you employ food to enhance your mood, the more likely it's that you are only going to get relief from feeling sick with addictive substances. Once we experience life's ups and downs with low tolerance, our primary coping mechanism is dopamine modification. Emotional imbalance results in excessive episodes of eating.

Starting Mindful Eating

You certainly already know: Naturally lean women have several properties that cause a healthy relationship with food:

- They only eat once they are physically hungry.
- They take the time to organize a healthy meal.
- They specialize in their eating experience and, if possible, eat silently.
- If possible, they dine in a pleasant place.
- They enjoy the food.
- They only take little bites.
- They often put their utensils down after each bite.
- They wholly and slowly chew the food.
- They breathe consciously before chewing the food.
- If food loses its taste, they stop eating immediately.

What is the idea of most of those habits? Eat mindfully. I used to always be intrigued when Naturally Thin Women used this phrase. But what's mindful eating? I wanted to understand what they did once they ate carefully. Use these four TCB steps to learn these practices of naturally thin women. Check them out:

- Recognize old patterns
- Interrupt the old pattern
- Perform NTW operation steps mindfully and with complete focus
- Measure progress and acknowledge success

Now we'll focus on each one of these practices of naturally thin women in a more detailed manner:

RECOGNIZING PHYSICAL HUNGER

Identify Starvation for the Situation

Five sorts of triggers instigate the current overeating programming. All of them are explained below:

- **Social Incentives:**

They eat to avoid feelings of inadequacy or to share a standard experience, hoping that it connects them to others. There's scientific evidence that we eat quite a lot when we dine in a social environment.

- **Sensual Trigger:**
  Eat for an opportunity, eat donuts at work, advertise food for food on TV, or when going by the bakery.
  I didn't feel the necessity to nourish my body, but I had the chance to experience joy and suddenly felt hungry. In these cases, the will to eat as a chance to experience the learned response, a pleasure to external triggers. We weren't hungry until we saw the visual food.
- **Motivational Trigger:**
  This means eating as a result of internal dialogue that condemns oneself. We offend ourselves, and ironically, succumbing to overeating usually reprimands us for lack of willpower.
- **Physiological Trigger:**
  Eating in response to a physical effect (e.g., headache or other pain).
- **Emotional Triggers:**
  Eating in response to boredom, stress, fatigue, tension, depression, anger, fear, and loneliness. These triggers are as simple as a scarcity of cognition within the body (I need a physical break) or as complex as suppressed emotions (I'm a member of a toxic

family).

Break the Obsession

My brain is crazy about food. I'm hungry and wired to feel obsessive about responding to food. Often my current wiring uses food counting on different situational triggers.

Name and Address Your Actual Needs

You have the choice of how to respond effectively to your triggers.

- **Social Trigger:**

To satisfy the desire to attach with others. I can try a couple of small bites and rave about the food. Even better, you'll start an exciting conversation about something aside from the menu.

- **TCB Answer:**

This is often not a pang of physical hunger. This is often my desire to adapt to society.

- **Sensual Trigger:**

Recognizing my usual reaction to the visual appeal of food. I admit I wasn't hungry before I saw the menu. We must assume that this is often not physical hunger; it's an automatic response to the unexpected.

- **TCB Answer:**

This is often not a pang of physical hunger. This is often my Pavlov's response to a highly charged stimulus. I would like to enjoy the pleasure that food provides. If I eat this, I will be able to feel better.

- **Motivational Trigger:**

Recognizing the standard reaction to negative thoughts, pain, and discomfort. Ending emotional stress may be a normal human reaction. I even have alternative and meaningful ways to affect feelings of inadequacy.

- **TCB Answer:**

This is often not a pang of physical hunger. Eating may be a way for me to settle down and the way I weaken my painful thoughts.

I even have the tools or can get the assistance I want to affect the painful dialogue inside.

- **Physiological Trigger:**

  There are simpler tools (medication as needed) to affect physical complaints.

- **TCB Answer:**

  This is often not a pang of physical hunger. This is often a learned reaction to physical illness.

- **Emotional Trigger:**

  You'll identify what triggers your emotional hunger and prefer to act effectively.

- **TCB Answer:**

This is often not physical hunger. That's my standard coping mechanism and current wiring.

Measure Progress

What about after performing steps 1–3? The scales within the Step 4 - Measures of Progress and knowledge of the Success section will assist you in measuring progress as you adopt individual characteristics. The more you practice, the better it'll be.

Is it possible for you to reply to every signal appropriately? If there is no solution, what's your stress level? Have you got to reduce stress first? What are the decisions that will satisfy your actual needs?

TAKE TIME TO PREPARE A HEALTHY MEAL

Home cooking has many advantages because it is a sort of mindfulness. You choose top quality and nutritious ingredients. Keep in mind that grocery stores are also stocked with cheap fats and cheap carbohydrates that don't offer you any nutritional value. You're controlling where your calories come from: whether that is from trans fats, additional sugars, or healthy vegetables. Make sure that there are not any flavor enhancers like MSG or other brain-disrupting substances.

Think about it; you've got to eat carefully.

The main way that can be achieved 95% of the time is through the quality of the food you eat. You do not know who is cooking your food or exactly what ingredients they use.

Are they cheap trans-fat oils with extra sodium and extra sugar? How can you put that in your body?

SITTING IN A BEAUTIFUL SETTING

Establish a natural and delightful environment to eat in, especially if you eat alone.

When you're hungry, it can take a couple of minutes to set up a beautiful setting. If you do not have the time, are in a hurry, and need to eat directly from the fridge, this is a warning sign that you're usually eating foods under high levels of stress. This might feel impossible while restoring your naturally lean female neural network. But it is important to heal the "hungry brain" and be calm before eating. There are several ways to scale back high levels of stress like deep breathing, meditation, journaling, active jogging, and anything that seems effective in reaching a state of peace. Remember to live your progress. Are you able to sit at the table without fear? If not, could you identify and explain your anxiety and address it?

EATING EXPERIENCE

In a culture that emphasizes multitasking, eating may be a secondary activity. We don't combine food with the nutrition of our bodies. Consumption is what we do without paying attention while doing more meaningful work.

Have you automatically turned off your car radio while trying to find a replacement address?

I instinctively know that removing a voice stimulus increases your ability to focus on finding an address. Silence also allows us to concentrate only on food and to be fully present for a dining experience.

Watching TV, interacting with computers, talking on the phone, reading books, and doing other activities isn't conducive to a careful diet. Mindful meals require indiscriminate attention, so it is a good way to overeat.

If you've got resistance to silent eating, rewiring can assist you in recognizing that you simply ate for the first time once you had another activity. It's a custom that has been cultivated for several years. You rarely focus on eating.

When you sit quietly and eat, you'll hear inner conversations, stop to enjoy the meal, and notice subtle messages from the body once you are satisfied. If turning off competing stimuli creates fear, inhale, and note the explanation for the anxiety.

If you're dining together with your family, invite them to participate in the careful process of eating. Try to recognize the distractions present during your meal; it is better than multitasking. Discuss your senses and taste of food. Slow eating doesn't need to be extreme. Nevertheless, it's a realistic idea to remind your family that eating isn't a race. Encourage your family to chew on every bite of food, examining the taste, texture, and smell intimately.

Ask them about their feelings, thank them for preparing this meal and give thanks and blessings for this time together to share a meal.

Remember to live your progress: how does one feel in silence after a meal? Are you able to eliminate all distractions and eat quietly without fear? Is practicing this strategy and eating silently getting easier?

ENJOY YOUR MEAL

Of course, the skinny women have an indoor dialogue of appreciation and acknowledgment and joy: "This is delicious. And you can really taste each herb"." Shoveling food not only misses every bite of taste but lacks the whole point of eating. You will need quality food to satisfy gourmet foodies because they need to be inspired by it.

We acknowledge that this resistance to internal dialogue is because of the current practice of not eating for the pleasure of eating. Usually, our conversation feeds on something aside from our body, so it's more relevant to issues, concerns, and current to-do lists.

If you pay 100% attention to eating and soak in the experience of eating carefully, you'll find that the restoration of the "naturally thin women's" wiring is approaching.

Remember to live your progress. How does one feel after allowing an indoor dialogue about the pleasure of eating?

Does one enjoy this conversation without fear? If the solution is not any, what are the obstacles to achieving this trait?

SMALL BITES

If you overeat food, you'll need to burn more calories but get the same amount of pleasure. We must recognize that we've made significant efforts in the past. The wise action is to eat some meals with a little spoon or child utensils while we learn to require smaller bites.

However, once you measure your progress during this area, it's essential to go back to normal-sized bites. The rationale is that if you're taking little bites simply because the spoon is small, the neural network won't be restored, and you're entirely hooked into the tool.

Don't forget to measure your progress. How do you feel after eating the entire meal with just a couple of bites? How was your fear? Did you experience pleasure with such a little amount? Did you want to run to the kitchen and obtain a more oversized spoon? Or did you start eating with your fingers?

CHEW SLOWLY AND THOROUGHLY

For many obsessive eaters, diet represents an answer similar to that of drug users. The faster you move the shovel, the quicker you rise.

Unfortunately, this behavior results in total calorie overload and shortens the feeling of delight. We want to raise our dopamine levels as soon as possible! We've been doing this for a long time, so chewing slowly and patiently is often a very anxious process.

The digestion begins with the first bite, which causes the discharge of saliva, disinfects food, and smooths the food on its way to the stomach.

As we chew, the brain releases neurotransmitters that tell the hypothalamus that we are full. Chewing slowly and deliberately will remove even the slightest aroma and increase your enjoyment.

Remember to live your progress. How does one feel after chewing slowly? What was your fear? Are you able to enjoy slowing down without fear?

BREATHING

After swallowing, breathing three times will reconnect you with your body. It's a sort of palate cleanser, if you like! Readjusting for each subsequent bite creates a sensual experience. This is also a chance to determine if we are full.

Remember to live your progress. Do you breathe three times after one bite? Did you notice that your anxiety is growing? Did you enjoy your meal?

EXPERIENCE FULLNESS

If you eat your food carefully, you will be full and be able to taste it! Don't rely on salt, ketchup, mayo, mustard, sugar, or barbecue sauces to create taste. Soon you will be able to regain the full experience and "enjoy" your food. Additives are an effort to nullify the knowledge that tells you that you simply have had enough.

Note that the start of this process feels strange. After all, we don't want to consume everything on the plate. For several folks, discarding food is extremely difficult because our conditioning to eat everything on the plate is deeply rooted. A useful tactic is to see excess food as fat in your favorite body parts. Your taste will tell you that this is ok, but overconsumption just means extra fat.

Also, understand that we are familiar with stomach congestion and not food consumption. Initially, this is often done mechanically, but if you repeat this a couple of times, you get the required saturation. Besides, regaining the confidence of your palate will make you feel free, as you will not get to experience the severity of a clogged sensation after a meal. The energy and satisfaction after eating, instead of lethargy or immobility, will make you regain your sense of freedom.

Remember to live your progress. Are you able to say, "it was great" and "I'm full" without having to stuff yourself? Are you ready to recognize the abundance?

3

Hypnosis

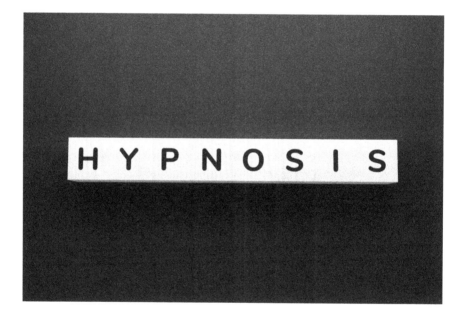

What Is Hypnosis?

Hypnosis is the act of leading someone to a state of trance. Various experts describe the trance state differently, but almost always, it includes:

- A deep state of relaxation.
- Hyper-focus and concentration.
- Increased suggestibility.

This may sound familiar. Many of us periodically go into and out of the trance state. You are in a trance state when you have zoned out when driving familiar roads, fallen into reverie while listening to music, or find yourself lost in a book or movie universe.

The only difference between hypnosis and this daily trance is that in hypnosis, someone causes the trance to accomplish something: recovery, exploration, or relief from stress, for instance.

What Is Hypnotherapy?

Consider hypnosis as a technique and hypnotherapy as the use of a method to explain the difference between hypnosis and hypnotherapy. SAT refers to hypnotherapy as art therapy in practice.

Hypnotherapy is clearly defined by the word itself. Hypnotherapy is the clinical form of hypnosis.

If you are a licensed psychiatrist or psychologist who uses hypnosis to help a patient resolve an emotional or physical disorder, you practice hypnotherapy.

The hypnotic trance is a surprisingly versatile instrument for addressing psychological and physical health problems. Here are just a few examples of using hypnotherapy for mental health and medical professionals:

Help people avoid smoking or alcohol abuse by concentrating their minds and promoting healthy behavior.

Establishing a connection between mind and body to alleviate chronic and acute pain, including surgery and birth. Hypnotherapy has also been shown to be effective against persistent physical disorders such as irritable bowel syndrome and dermatologic disorders.

Immerse yourself in the subconscious mind to identify and treat the root causes of mental health problems like depression, anxiety, PTSD, and addiction. We will concentrate on this last use for the rest of this essay. The trance state is the secret to revealing hidden layers in our minds, memories, and intentions, as many hypnotherapists have figured out.

Does Hypnotherapy Work? What Does the Science Say?

Since it allows direct access to the subconscious mind, hypnotherapy is more effective than conventional recovery approaches for many therapists.

"Hypnotherapy helps us to slip under the logical part of our mind," says Stacie Beam-Bruce, a hypnotherapist. "We can't understand why we do something or why we feel something because it doesn't make sense. Hypnotherapy has access to the emotional convictions of trauma."

We recently spoke to 23 qualified hypnotherapists, and everyone said that hypnotherapy had changed their practice and the lives of their clients. In our free e-book, you can read their stories.

But there is more than anecdotal evidence of the workings of hypnotherapy.

"While hypnosis has been controversial, most clinicians now accept that it can be a strong, efficient medical technique for a wide range of conditions, such as pain, anxiety, and mood disorders." The American Psychological Association concludes.

In 2001 a working group was commissioned by the British Psychological Society to review the evidence and to create a comprehensive report on hypnotherapy. "An array of research has now been accumulated to show that the use of hypnotic approaches may be useful for handling and treating a wide variety of medical, psychological, and psychotherapeutic problems."

Modern brain imaging technology now provides us with a panorama of hypnotherapy's physical manifestations. Stanford researchers found that parts of the brain correlated with understanding and improvement showed "changed behavior and connectivity" while analyzing the brains of 57 individuals undergoing hypnosis.

How Can You Be Trained in Hypnotherapy?

Hypnotherapy is a strong, scientifically proven resource to help your clients enter their unconscious minds and solve their most difficult mental health problems.

But there are other practical reasons to perform hypnotherapy training as a licensed psychotherapist.

We also found, in a recent market survey, that hypnotherapists can easily make six figures from their practice annually. For an effective hypnotherapy service, here are a few other things to keep in mind:

- Charge more for extra services.
- Only recommend other providers sparingly.
- Think hard about joining an insurance panel.
- Begin your private practice in a market that is not saturated.

How are you going to learn hypnotherapy, then? There is no clear route to certification for hypnotherapy, but we suggest staying away from solo teachers. They typically lack the teaching experience or the network that exists with a college or vocational school.

Find an alternative for hypnotherapy training that:

- Is valid for ongoing training loans.
- Offers certification results (especially relevant for the reimbursement of insurance).
- Is taught by teachers with real expertise in clinical hypnotherapy.
- Incorporates realistic instruction.

History of Hypnosis

The earliest hypnosis references come from ancient Egypt and Greece. In reality, 'Hypnos' refers to the god and is the Greek word for sleep, while hypnosis is very different from sleep. Both cultures had religious centers where people came for help to their problems. Hypnosis was used to trigger hallucinations and then studied to get to the root of the problem. Within early literature, there are also references to trance and hypnosis. In 2600 BC in China, Wong Tai wrote about techniques involving incantations and hand passes. Hypnotic procedures were also described by the Hindu Vedas written around 1500 BC. In many shamanic, druid, audio, yogic and religious practices, trance-like states occur frequently.

Hypnosis' modern father was an Austrian doctor, Franz Mesmer (1734–1815), from whose name comes the word 'mesmerism.' Despite being poorly maligned by his day's medical world, Mesmer was nevertheless a brilliant man. He developed the 'animal magnetism' theory—the idea that disease is a result of blockages in the flow of magnetic forces within the body.

He felt he might preserve his animal magnetism in iron filings baths and transmit it to patients with rods or 'mesmeric passes.'

The mesmeric pass certainly must go down in history as one of the most interesting and certainly the longest-winded ways to get someone into a trance. Mesmer was standing still for his subjects while he was sweeping his arms over their bodies, sometimes for hours. I suspect that the effect of boring patients into a trance was probably quite amusing, but it certainly was effective. Mesmer himself was a showman who made the patient feel like anything could happen. This form of indirect suggestion was quite powerful in itself. Mesmer was also responsible for the presentation of hypnotizing man, with magnetic eyes, a cap, and a goat's bar. His popularity sparked envy among many of his colleagues, contributing to his public humiliation. Looking back, it is somewhat unbelievable that hypnosis survived its early years since the scientific community was set against it.

John Elliotson (1791–68), a professor at London University, who was famous for bringing the stethoscope to England, was also a progressive thinker. He also tried to defend the use of mesmerism but had to resign. Within his own home, he managed to show mesmerism for all interested parties, contributing to a gradual increase within the literature.

In the mid-19th century, James Braid (1795–1860) was the next true founder of hypnosis in Great Britain.

He developed an interest in mesmerism by chance, primarily through a Scottish eye doctor. One day when he was late for an appointment, in the waiting room, he found his patient staring at an old lamp with his eyes sparkling. Fascinated, Braid ordered the patient to close his eyes and go to sleep. The patient was pleased with the "therapy," and the interest in hypnotherapy for Braid grew. He found that the willingness of a patient is one of the most critical components to get them into a trance.

The Swinging Watch, which is associated with hypnosis by many people, was a common fixation object in the early days. Braid published a book after his discovery that the palaver of mesmeric passes was not necessary. He suggested that the process now be referred to as hypnotism.

In the meantime, James Esdaile (1808–59), a British surgeon in India, recognized the immense benefits of hypnotic pain relief and conducted hundreds of major operations using hypnotism as the only anesthetic. Once he returned to England, he tried to explain his results to the medical authorities, but they laughed at him and proclaimed hypnotism ineffective (they preferred modern chemical anesthetics, which they could regulate and charge more money for, of course). Hypnosis has since been and remains an "alternative" form of treatment.

The French were also interested in the hypnosis issue, and numerous breakthroughs were made by men like Ambrose Liébeault (1823–1904), J.M. Charcot (1825–93), and Charles Richet (1850–1935), respectively.

The work of Émile Coué (1857–1926), another Frenchman, was quite important. He stepped away from traditional methods and allowed the use of autosuggestion pioneers. He is best known for writing, "Day by day I get better and better in every way." His approach was one of encouragement and has been championed in countless modern books.

A man of great kindness, Coué believed that he didn't cure people himself but that he helped them to cure themselves. He recognized how important the involvement of the subject was in hypnosis and was a precursor to modern practitioners who say, "There is no such thing as hypnosis; there is only self-hypnosis." For example, if you ask someone to pass through a wooden board on the ground, they can do so without wobbling. But if you tell them to close their eyes and think the board is suspended hundreds of feet above ground between two buildings, they start to swing.

In some ways, Coué also predicted the placebo effect—medication of no inherent value that stills helps patients that are offered a drug that will heal them. Recent placebo research is quite shocking.

Statistics sometimes show that placebos can work better than many of the most popular drugs in modern medicine.

Although drugs are not always necessary to recover from disease, there seems to be a conviction of recovery.

Sigmund Freud (1856–1939) also took an interest in hypnosis and used it at first. He eventually gave up on the practice—mostly because he wasn't very good at it for several reasons! He preferred psychoanalysis, which involved a lot of listening to the patient lying on a sofa. He felt the evolution of the self was a complicated process that progressed through phases of sexual development, with the main cause of psychological disorders being repressed memories of traumatic events. This is an interesting idea that still needs to be demonstrated.

Freud's early rejection of hypnosis hindered the growth of hypnotherapy, shifting the therapeutic focus away from hypnosis and into psychoanalysis. However, in the 1930s, the publication of Clark Hull's book 'Hypnosis and Suggestibility' shook things up in America.

Previously, Milton H. Erickson, MD (1901–80), a remarkable man and a highly skilled psychotherapist, became the acknowledged leading expert in clinical hypnosis. He was disabled and diagnosed with polio since he was a teenager, but he never let that stop him.

He had an exceptional opportunity to observe people when paralyzed, and he noticed that what people said and did was very different.

He was fascinated by human psychology and developed several innovative and creative ways of healing people. He used metaphors, surprise, uncertainty, laughter, and hypnosis to heal. A master of 'indirect hypnosis,' he was able to place a person in a trance without even using the word hypnosis.

It is now accepted that recognizing hypnosis is necessary for the efficient exercise of all kinds of psychotherapy. Erickson's approach and its derivatives are the most effective techniques without any doubt.

Over the years, hypnosis in the medical profession has evolved and become more respectable. Although hypnosis and medicine are not the same, they are now recognized as related, and it is only a matter of time before hypnosis becomes a common practice acceptable to the public as much as a dentist's visit.

General Benefits of Hypnosis

STOP SMOKING

When you try to find the perfect way to quit smoking, you'll find most options come with a long list of over-the-counter and prescription-nicotine-replacement medications and non-nicotine prescriptions.

NO MORE OVEREATING

Healthier food choices and exercise are the main things required for weight loss, but effective weight loss in some situations often requires eliminating emotional and unconscious factors that keep us from losing weight.

SLEEP BETTER

Failure to sleep can impair memory and decision making, which can lead to chronic health issues, including heart disease, obesity, and depression. Although there are several therapies for insomnia, including medicine, exercise, and cognitive therapy, hypnotherapy also works exceptionally well.

EASE CHRONIC PAIN

Pain is a signal which helps us realize something is wrong. But in chronic pain, even after the body is healed, the nervous system can still relay the pain signal.

MANAGE BEREAVEMENT

The death of a loved one can create a sense of loss or sorrow that may weaken your ability to control impulses, trigger anxiety, insomnia, and depression.

When you are going through loss, crying can help your mind and body register what is happening. Mental Health America and the American Psychological Association also recommend dealing with loss by processing the death of a loved one, taking care of your health, reaching out to others who have experienced loss, acknowledging your emotions, and working towards enjoying the life you have now. The loss management mechanisms are personal. Hypnotherapy helps to cope with signs of grief by offering constructive thoughts and trying to find ways of coping with loss over time. Some experts help people cope with loss by putting a "timer" on their sorrow. "Normally, when they are sick and tired of sickness and tired of grief, they let me know," says Barker.

RELIEVE ANXIETY

Anyone that has dealt with anxiety can understand how the condition can become worse and turn desperate. Anxiety disorders are the most prevalent in psychiatric illnesses affecting more than 25 million Americans, according to the American Psychiatric Association. Although fear is typically treated by medicine or therapy or by a combination of both, many people are also turning to hypnotherapy. A hypnotist aims to determine whether the anxiety is due to psychological, physical, or other factors.

STOP TINNITUS

Sounds that no one except you can detect is a symptom of tinnitus, a disease that 45 million Americans have encountered, according to the American Tinnitus Association, like ringing, moaning, or whistling.

While tinnitus can be temporary or long-lasting, most forms of the disorder are not healed. Recovery methods include visual aids, behavior therapy, sound therapy, and TMJ therapy. Hypnosis is an alternative, too. "Tinnitus is caused by the mind," Barker says. "It's because the individual expects it to happen, and the sound goes away until you get rid of the thought of waiting for it."

MAKE CHEMOTHERAPY MORE TOLERABLE

One of the earliest known applications of cancer hypnosis occurred in 1829. Doctor Chapelain used hypnosis to alleviate a breast cancer patient's pain. The doctor used hypnosis as an anesthetic during mastectomy and surgery, while the patient was said to be "calm and showed good pain control." While the standard procedure for surgery today is anesthesia, hypnosis still plays a role in cancer care and is often used to relieve tension and anxiety and alleviate side effects of chemotherapeutics such as nausea and vomiting. "We help you mainly cope with your symptoms and encourage you to improve how you handle pain," said Woods, who deals mostly with cancer patients. "We cannot give them false hope, but we can place them safely and encourage them to heal." She says that cancer patients are sometimes moved from doctor to doctor, and they feel like they are just a number for them.

"We monitor our customers during their chemotherapy appointment, which is a personal encounter with a hypnotherapist that can take a long time."

IMPROVE ATHLETIC PERFORMANCE

Michael Jordan, Tiger Woods, and Mike Tyson are only some well-known athletes who have turned to hypnosis in their athletic success.

Athletes started using hypnosis long ago to remove negative emotions, de-stress and calm the mind and body and improve concentration so that they can 'stay in the field.' The therapy will enhance confidence, discipline, and ability and extends to all levels of athletes, including those who are recovering from injury and those who are just getting started. Most athletes go to a hypnotist to improve performance, but they end up improving their minds.

EASE IBS

The International Federation for Functional Diseases reports that irritable bowel syndrome (IBS) affects 25 to 45 million people in the US. Although the exact cause of IBS is not known, the impact of the disease may vary from mild to weakening. Stress can worsen IBS symptoms, although it is not the cause of it. Although medication varies from probiotics to diets that reduce food triggering—such as low-FODMAP diet—to antidepressants and cognitive behavioral therapy, hypnosis has also been shown to be an effective treatment of IBS in research. Hypnotherapy uses methods of relaxation and hypnotic suggestions to help patients manage their symptoms. The results of the studies showed that the quality of life and frequent symptoms of abdominal pain, constipation, diarrhea, and bloating improve for most patients.

IMMUNE SYSTEM RESPONSE

Taking care of your immune system and controlling it is simpler than you think. You might ask yourself, "Is your immune system influenced?" You're going to be glad to learn it is.

Most people today understand that the effect of stress on our immune system is negative. They are more likely to become ill and take longer to recover from long-term stress than people who have less stressful lives if they deal with long-term stress. Stress is anticipated in our modern world. Stress management strategies and relaxation protocols can significantly affect your immune system's health.

Hypnosis is also an effective method for controlling stress and anxiety every day. As you can deal with everyday pressures and problems better, your immune system gets stronger and helps protect weaker parts of the body.

When we relax, the brain releases endorphins to restore the balance of hormones, to control the nervous system, and to encourage a balanced immune system.

INFERTILITY

Yes, hypnotherapy can help you with infertility. Yes, it's real.

In the United States, about 6.1 million couples are trying to conceive, and it can take a year or more for most people to get pregnant. But it can take much longer for others.

When we plan to start a family and get pregnant, it's always a burden and a worry to get nothing in every mind. Our mind starts to generate all sorts of excuses and causes women to try and Google, "Why don't I get pregnant?!" The more irritated, depressed, or worried you get, the stress hormones your body frees will make it even less likely that you will conceive easily.

It's like your body wants you to be calm and able to embrace the responsibility that you ask for before it takes place. Hypnotherapy may be an ideal alternative or complementary treatment to allow you to feel confident and ready to have a baby. Hypnosis will help you to feel more confident, relaxed, and handle stress better every day.

This prevents the body from releasing adrenaline and cortisol hormones into the bloodstream. Too much of these hormones can make it difficult to conceive as they interfere with the brain portion that regulates other hormones.

The stress of infertility will also reduce Dad's level of testosterone and the consistency of semen, making the whole thing much more complicated for you both.

Hypnotherapy can resolve fertility issues by helping both mother and dad to feel calmer, more relaxed, and controlled, and thereby reduce stress and anxiety.

SEASONAL AND FOOD ALLERGIES

Hypnosis is a highly effective (no side effects) remedy in the fight against environmental and food allergies. Allergies in springtime, such as hay fever, are caused by an acute reaction or allergic pollen reaction. Hay fever (like any allergy) is an immune system overreaction. The immune system wrongly identifies the pollen as a threat and produces an unwanted reaction.

Hypnosis and Hypnotherapy

Hypnosis and hypnotherapy are often described as being in the same practice, but they are not.

Hypnotherapy is a type of guided hypnosis that mainly focuses on concentration, while hypnosis guides an individual into a trance state of mind. With hypnosis, this state is commonly referred to as either a resting state of relaxation, induced suggestibility, or hyper-focus.

Something the average student or individual working battles with daily is to keep focus during their daily routine.

A consistent lack of focus may leave an individual feeling tired, unmotivated, stressed, and inefficient. That's just one of the main reasons why hypnotherapy serves as the ultimate solution for anyone looking to improve productivity, relieve stress and anxiety, and boost overall health.

Hypnotherapy is used in various instances, all of which have been proven to be very effective. It is similar to other types of psychological treatments with benefits that are similar to those of psychotherapy.

The practice treats conditions, including phobias, anxiety disorders, bad habits, weight gain, substance abuse, learning disorders, poor communication skills, and can even treat pain.

It can resolve digestive and gastrointestinal disorders, and severe hormonal skin disorders, aiding as a massive solution to many different issues people face daily and are often unaware of how to treat them.

Many patients with immune disorders or severe conditions, such as cancer, can also be treated with hypnotherapy, known for its pain-relieving abilities. It is especially helpful and used when patients undergo chemotherapy or physical rehabilitation that is excessively painful.

Hypnotherapy is carried out by a therapist in a therapeutic and tranquil environment that allows them to enter and remain in a focused state of mind.

Apart from its incredible benefits, it can adjust the mind and shift mental behavior, almost tricking the brain into focusing on positive intentions. Often, with severe cases, such as advanced stages of cancer, patients are almost convinced that they are not going to live very long. Some may even receive their expected date of passing from their medical practitioner.

Faced with extreme negativity, such as a patient being told that they are going to die, patients tend to give up.

Now, regardless of what will happen, what your mind conceives to believe may very well become a reality.

This manner of thinking holds a lot of truth and could set a patient apart from surviving their condition. Although it is difficult to achieve a state of mind where one is positive when faced with illness, hypnotherapy can indeed adjust one's thought process and retrain the brain into thinking only positive thoughts.

In essence, a cancer patient's attitude can massively contribute to their probability of healing.

Hypnotherapy can relieve not only pain but also add a mental shield against negative thinking processes that could contribute to a patient's inability to recover.

From various types of recovery, acting as more than just a supportive release for pain, emotional and mental stability, something many individuals find fascinating is that one can lose weight with hypnotherapy.

Depending on the severity of the problem being treated, hypnotherapy may take longer to see a difference. Upon meeting with a hypnotherapist, the practitioner will assess the extent of hypnotherapy required, measured in hours, for the patient to obtain the result they would like to see at the end of their course of therapy. A specific total number of hours will be prescribed to the patient, forming a part of alternative healthcare.

Take it as a tip; with hypnotherapy, it is very important to feel comfortable with your practitioner, which is why you must seek out several to find the right one. With hypnotherapy, it's always a good idea to ask around for recommendations and not settle for the first therapist you come across.

Since you now have a good understanding of hypnotherapy, it's necessary also to be informed about hypnosis.

Hypnosis refers to placing an individual in a trance state of mind, also referred to as deep relaxation, increased suggestibility, and hyperfocus.

Thinking about the different references related to hypnosis, one may think of it as being focused on deep sleep. When we sleep, we tend to enter and exit a trance state quite often. This can also occur when we listen to music or when we are focused on reading a book or watching a movie. It invites a state of mind where our thought processes almost come to a halt as we are focused, and our brain is quieter than it is used to.

Whenever you immerse yourself in something and focus, you enter a trance state of mind.

So, what's the difference between professional hypnosis, induced hypnosis, and our brief everyday moments of intense focus?

Well, the only difference is that with hypnosis, you are assisted by a hypnotherapist to enter a trance state of mind where you can achieve wonderful things. You can achieve a state of motivation, positivity, healing, stress-relief, and even weight loss.

THE MYTHS

Those who believe in myths or are superstitious have painted a picture of hypnosis that has managed to scare people away.

Whether you've heard about hypnosis in the media, saw it in a movie, or were shunned by your parents against learning more about it, you can rest assured that it's not as bad as society makes it out to be.

Can hypnotists control the minds of their patients? Of course not. Hypnosis is used as a medical practice to either relieve symptoms associated with pain or anxiety or help people lose weight and get back on the healthy train again. It doesn't leave you feeling helpless or unaware of what you're doing.

During hypnotherapy, patients are still conscious and can hear everything that is happening around them, which is why it is considered an entirely safe practice. To assure people even more, it is next to impossible for anyone to be unconscious when undergoing hypnosis.

Differentiating between hypnosis and hypnotherapy, you now have learned that both practices have a similar foundation and can help patients achieve different goals. Both practices can indeed help patients lose weight.

When you want to lose weight, you have to focus on different things. Losing weight is never just about cleaning up your diet and incorporating exercise into your daily routine.

Since stress is a major part of the reason our bodies hold onto weight, hypnosis serves as the perfect solution to relieve stress and can also manage disorders, often contributing to weight gain. This includes both anxiety and depression. Also, it can help individuals with either an overactive or underactive thyroid reach some balance level, allowing one's body to lose weight permanently and sustainably.

Hypnotherapy, on the other hand, is perfect for treating many different cases, including bad habits like smoking and overeating, which can contribute to a variety of eating disorders. Both can help you develop a bad relationship with food and even act as a means of coping with stress.

That is why hypnosis and hypnotherapy can work hand-in-hand to achieve attainable results, depending on your needs. Hypnotherapy also relieves mind-body illnesses and reduces symptoms, including irritable bowel syndrome, skin conditions, and various addictions.

Unless you suffer from severe stress-related disorders that require you to engage in both practices, hypnotherapy can serve all of your needs concerning weight loss. It is the perfect option for anyone aiming to achieve long-term results.

Given that every decision, thought, and intention is birthed in the brain, it's quite simple to see why hypnotherapy can solve a lot of the problems we as humans face with our bodies today.

Both hypnosis and hypnotherapy serve as practices that help deplete negative habits and can assist anyone, no matter how sick or unmotivated, to get back on track, follow a healthy diet, and available exercise program, as well as kick many harmful addictions.

Working Principles of Hypnosis

Any kind of hypnosis, whether it is guided or self-induced, works by bypassing the conscious critical faculty and accessing the subconscious mind. Therefore, in order to understand how hypnosis works, we need to first discuss how the subconscious mind is structured and what its functions are.

We have two regions of the mind; the aware portion and what we term the "subconscious." There are somewhat specific functions between these two sections.

For example, after you cut your finger, you may deliberately plan to wash the injury and add a plaster. But the subconscious manages the entire job that actually repairs the cut. The development of an inflamed region protects the remainder of the skin against contamination, the immune response kills off the infection, and the body produces fresh skin to cover what was destroyed—so all that occurs without any cognitive feedback! When we speak about hypnosis and hypnotherapy, we also apply it to the subconscious mind.

The strength of this "invisible" portion of our consciousness is beyond doubt. The subconscious controls our every waking minute, deciding the individuals we want, how we respond to others, our habits of action in different circumstances, the stuff we "cannot bear at any expense," the kind of entertainment we like, our sexual behaviors and everything we do is at minimum influenced, if not regulated, by our subconscious mechanisms. In reality, the subconscious mind does not think. The subconscious is absolute without justification or reasoning, criticism or judgment, approval, or consent. Anything in the subconscious is black or white; either it is, or it is not. It is, in essence, nothing but a responsive psychological hub where our intuitive powers live, those with which we were born and those which we have gained over the life span.

For every split second in our lives, it is an appraisal device that continually measures every single input through our sensory experiences.

The subconscious interacts only through thoughts with rational awareness. So, it utilizes the contact to try and keep us safe. It seems like any new feedback from the five senses can be measured against what we have seen so far in our existence. Whether the new feedback fits something that has already been done, so the response that we have will focus on the outcome, be it a positive response, which may be enjoyment, or a negative reaction that may be anxiety. The subconscious processes are largely unseen. The subconscious becomes utterly inaccessible to awareness. Obviously, no person can sense his or her subconscious at work because we don't have some way to tell what the latest feedback is really being correlated with, which accounts for why we may unexpectedly hate a particular individual or even encounter a burst of anxiety for any fairly small occurrence. Of course, it can function in reverse almost as easily; have you ever had a case when you want to have something so much that it sometimes confuses you? Then you wind up doing things like: "God knows why I'm so stuck on this." This may be a peculiarly offensive friend, or maybe a clothing item or almost anything.

The subconscious is extremely quick in its capacity to interpret.

Now it's a little difficult to take on board, but it's a reality that by the time you become fully aware of a stimulus, a signal from all of the senses, even your own thinking processes, the subconscious has detected it, checked it many thousand times, and already planned an action. But the thinking mind gets in the way, and that's the root of tension in a nutshell. The subconscious mind might encourage you to undertake an activity that is separate from what you actively intend to do.

The amygdala does not respond to intentional thinking. The truth about the unconscious is that it does not allow us the ability to actively think our way into what it does, as it interacts with us simply through emotions that control our reactions. When we seek to resolve certain feelings and emotions through rational thinking, the subconscious doubles its attempts! Have you ever attempted to stop feeling anxious because the thinking mind is unable to understand that there is anxiety in the first place? Public speaking is an outstanding illustration of that sort of stuff. Most individuals have unreasonable public-speaking anxiety, but what would really happen after all? Okay, you could make a mistake and maybe miss what you were about to say. But the dry mouth, leg-shaking, stomach-churning, heart-pumping sensation of true panic that can occur in just talking about it is a little 'over-the-top,' if viewed rationally! Yet this doesn't help at all even when you know it.

Hypnosis helps one to connect with the subconscious. Once the cycle occurs in our subconscious, it's always futile striving to force the shift in our conscious mind.

Hypnosis helps one create positive improvements in the very roots of our subconscious—and even so, it can be a profoundly incredible force for good. By accessing the state of hypnosis, we can easily circumvent the portion of the mind of the Conscious Critical Faculty and 'rewire' the subconscious so that it accepts fresh, new ideas. Hypnosis is something that anyone will profit from. When you notice that you do things you don't want to do regularly or consistently don't do anything you need/would like to do, then you're mentally unwell; that is, you have a sign. Often though, a symptom is nothing but the manifestation of the idea that the subconscious has learned something that is in disagreement with conscious expectations or needs. Hypnosis and hypnotherapy encourage one to find a way to circumvent or shine a light on this latent thought and either re-examine its relevance or use suggestions to make it dormant.

Due to its effectiveness, hypnosis appears to be prescribed for just about anything: from avoiding smoking to weight reduction to alcohol abuse. Evidence shows hypnosis is an effective self-improvement device. Hypnotherapy operates by encouraging patients to alter ingrained values and upgrade them.

Using hypnosis, we re-frame and revise old ideas—why, for example, stopping smoking would be challenging and unpleasant—and replacing them with new, more effective beliefs.

Here's a simple way to explain hypnotherapy: hypnosis is a mental condition of extreme calm in which we skip the conscious mind. That is to say; the mind is calm and able to learn; the subconscious is even more open to suggestion.

Here's an example: Assume you choose to use hypnosis to lose weight. Your subconscious mind retains several assumptions regarding weight loss. You may assume automatically: It's hard to lose weight, you don't want to give up your comfort snacks, or you don't have time to work out. Ultimately, these implicit beliefs—formed by images, interactions, and perceptions—guide our deliberate behavior, and we don't really know that it is happening. In essence, our subconscious is setting us up for disappointment. So that's representative of all of our poor habits—negative self-talk, drinking, overeating—all of which are profoundly ingrained in subconscious thought.

Nonetheless, by hypnosis, we can start modifying and reviewing these detrimental beliefs. So this may clarify why the literature clearly indicates that hypnosis operates with problems such as chronic pain, abuse of drugs, and losing weight.

Through teaching our minds to think about problems and aspirations differently, we will eradicate the negative thinking, which too often contributes to self-sabotage. Hypnosis, as mentioned, allows you to alter your unwanted thinking. And this is how hypnosis works, in a nutshell.

4

Self-Hypnosis

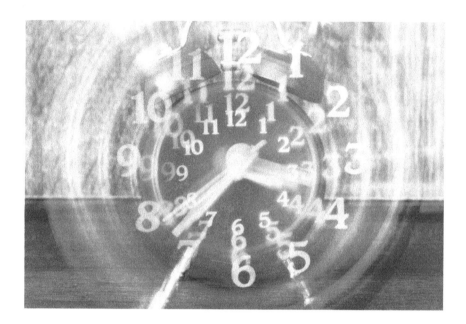

What Is Self-Hypnosis?

Self-hypnosis is, like hypnosis, an altered state of consciousness that is halfway between waking and sleeping. It is characterized by a decrease in the activity of the functions of our conscious part and an increased activity of the unconscious functions.

Unlike Ericksonian hypnosis, there is no need to be guided by a therapist to practice self-hypnosis: it can be done without outside help, even if it is advisable to follow a few introductory sessions with a practitioner.

Hypnosis is an effective and accessible means for everyone to get in touch with their unconscious. Like hypnosis in a therapist's office, it is practiced regularly (it is up to you to define the frequency) having before defined a session objective: stop smoking, snacking, reduce stress or anxiety whatever the goal you choose, regular self-hypnosis has many physical and mental health benefits.

Indeed, depending on the state of consciousness in which you find yourself, the brain emits waves of different frequencies.

The beta waves are faster, consistent with our normal operation in the standby state. At this frequency, we are intellectually available.

The slightly slower alpha waves are emitted when we are in a state of inner calm, without intellectual effort. They already correspond to a modified state of consciousness, which can be obtained simply by closing our eyes.

The theta waves are characterized by an even greater relaxation and correspond to our REM sleep.

Finally, the delta waves (the slowest) are emitted by our brains when we are in a deep sleep.

When we are in a hypnotic trance, our brain emits alpha waves. This cerebral rhythm is notably associated with:

- reduced anxiety
- improvement of sleep disorders
- reduction in blood pressure and heart rate
- increased levels of serotonin (a neurotransmitter responsible for regulating mood)

By increasing your production of alpha waves through the regular practice of self-hypnosis, you, therefore, ensure a state of relaxation favorable to better general health.

Self-hypnosis is a powerful method in which you talk at the subconscious mind or part of your brain. It gives you a way to eliminate any obstacles and confusion within the dialogue of your mind-body.

Self-hypnosis is still considered a mystical phenomenon by many people, even though this technique can be seen as prayer. You are alone, and you concentrate on your well-being. If you like, you ask God or a supreme being you believe in to help you. This practice also includes meditation (just like praying does), as well as chanting, mantras, inner confirmations, or affirmations. When you have to perform at work or college, you make such statements like "I don't fear; I'm fine"; "I can do it" or exactly the opposite, like "I can't do it. Everybody is better than me," etc. Even when we imagine ourselves in a different scenario from what is currently happening, we are programming ourselves. What you are doing is continuously hypnotizing yourself. Self-hypnosis helps us to come into contact with the unconscious through the use of specific language, aimed at awakening some parts of ourselves by leveraging archetypal symbols. Self-hypnotization is self-programming.

Our unconscious understands the symbolic messages of words rather than their rational meaning; that's why figurative language is used in hypnosis for inducing the individual to relax and to focus on the inner world.

We are embedding a vivid, information-rich image with emotions in the subconscious mind.

However, we must learn to pray, or let's say hypnotize ourselves accurately! Self-hypnosis is the ability to apply techniques and procedures alone to stimulate the unconscious to become our ally and involve it directly in the realization of our goals. By learning the essential elements of communication with the unconscious mind, it is possible to become able to reprogram activities of our unconscious. Self-hypnosis is a method that does not dismiss the support of a professional but has the advantage of being able to be performed independently. This is possible through the use of CDs and DIY courses made by hypnotists to make this practice accessible to a larger number of people with significant advantages, even from an economic point of view!

It is merely a process of moving variables; you become the inductee of the relaxed state and the one who suggests the positive ideas for change on yourself. You are both the guide into the relaxed state and the one experiencing the relaxed state.

While this might seem like it ups the ante and makes the process much more complicated just by increasing your number of roles and responsibilities, it is much simpler than you could ever imagine.

Basic Principles
CONSCIOUS AND UNCONSCIOUS

Like hypnosis, the practice of self-hypnosis rests on an optimistic vision of the unconscious. It is considered a reservoir of learning, skills, and creative solutions, from which you can draw to solve all kinds of problems. It is, therefore, an ally in the context of therapy and the achievement of your goals.

Unconscious thinking, which is emotional and symbolic, relates to our right hemisphere. However, daily, we connect mainly to our left hemisphere, responsible for our conscious part: this produces an analytical, rational, and discursive thought, which has been transmitted to us by education. It tends to obscure the unconscious part, which generates internal conflicts.

RESTORE THE BALANCE BETWEEN LEFT AND RIGHT BRAIN

The practice of hypnosis and self-hypnosis is based on the premise that most of our problems come from poor communication between the left brain and the right brain.

Most often, the left brain analyzes and categorizes what we are going through, and we consciously believe that a problem is solved. However, irrational behavior suggests the opposite: it is because the concern has not been resolved on an emotional and unconscious level.

Self-Hypnosis Techniques

Self-hypnosis involves putting yourself in a trance. There are several techniques for self-hypnotizing: at the start of your practice, you can try several to find the one that works best for you. Here are some examples of effective trance inductions to practice alone:

THE SENSE SPIRAL

This technique was developed by Betty Erickson, the wife of the famous psychiatrist and hypnotherapist Milton Erickson. It consists of stimulating all sensory perceptions to provoke a saturation (and therefore a relaxation) of the conscious mind.

First, focus your attention on a specific point at eye level or slightly above it. With your eyes open or closed, start by stating (aloud or in thought) 5 sentences that describe your visual experience ("I see..."); then five sentences describing your hearing experience ("I hear..."), then five sentences describing your kinaesthetic experience ("I feel...").

Then repeat the same sequence, but with 4 sentences, then 3, then 2, then only one per direction.

THE BODY SCAN

This inducing trance is inspired by yoga and Buddhist meditation.

Sitting or lying down, focus your attention successively on different parts of your body, starting from the top of the head to reach the feet.

Accompanying this movement and self-relaxation suggestions will allow you to relax each part of the body so you can finally reach a state of overall relaxation.

BREATHING

Again, this method is inspired by yoga and meditation techniques. With your eyes closed, focus on your breathing. Become aware of inhalation and expiration. The rhythm of your breathing will gradually decrease, which will allow you to enter quickly and naturally into a trance.

THE RESOURCE LANDSCAPE

This method consists of identifying a pleasant place attached to a pleasant or imagined memory.

With your eyes closed to facilitate visualization, take a path or a staircase that leads you to this place.

Once in this place, the idea is to immerse yourself in all the elements present: the images, the sounds, the physical sensations, possibly the smells. With training, it will become easier and easier for you to remember or imagine details.

ANCHORAGES

Anchoring is a very powerful hypnosis technique, which consists of associating an external stimulus (visual, auditory, or kinesthetic element) with an internal state of a given emotional response. The anchor is often used to counter addictions, for example, by associating with the sight of a glass of alcohol, an emotional reaction of disgust.

In self-hypnosis, anchors can be used to enter into a trance. For example, you can help yourself with a small object, a gesture, a smell, a sentence, or even a piece of music. By using the element of your choice at the start of each session, you will gradually condition yourself. So, you will end up naturally establishing an association between this stimulus and going into a trance. The success of the anchoring method depends mainly on its repetition.

INDICATIONS

There are many indications of self-hypnosis. Before each session, it is good to define a clear session objective. This objective can take the form:

- Of a mental state that you want to reach (inner, calm, self-confidence, letting go, absence of stress, and anxiety)
- A harmful behavior or habit from which you want to break away (cigarette addiction, snacking, procrastination)

- Of fears and other obstacles that you want to go beyond (phobias, fright, shyness)
- Of the performance that you want to enhance (athletic performance, cognitive ability, doing public speaking or sitting an exam)

How to Enter a State of Hypnotic Trance?

At the start of your practice, if you have difficulty self-hypnotizing yourself, several solutions are available. For example:

The use of professional audio recordings: you can buy them at very reasonable prices, online, in a CD, or in the form of downloadable mp3 files. Many hypnosis videos are also available for free on YouTube.

Getting help from a hypnotherapist is the most reliable way to get started. In the office, a practitioner teaches you the techniques and protocols best suited to your problem; you can then practice them at home.

Contraindications and Danger

Hypnosis and self-hypnosis are contraindicated for people suffering from dissociative mental illnesses (paranoia, schizophrenia, bipolar disorder). Indeed, hypnotic trance increases the risk of decompensating.

Apart from this particular case, the practice of self-hypnosis is harmless, provided that certain rules are respected, in particular:

- Practice in a quiet place where you are safe (a decrease in alertness accompanies the state of hypnosis)
  Put in place safety fuses, that is, affirmations that allow you to stay in control and have a good experience. For example: "I am going to live a positive and useful experience, from which I will wake up relaxed and full of energy."
  How to Self-Hypnotize for Weight Loss
  The procedure of hypnosis is getting your psyche into a state where it can acknowledge a proposal. During hypnosis, a subject

can bring profound new realizations into their inner mind to dispense with convictions and propensities that might be hindering their regular daily existence.

This is the reason why hypnosis is so well known for those trying to lose weight. In any case, it isn't imperative to look for and pay for a specialist. Most insurance plans don't take care of the cost of hypnotherapy, either. Attempt to self-entrance yourself to lose additional weight.

Stage 1

Schedule time in your day where other activities won't sidetrack you. Attempt to set aside at least a half-hour where you'll keep yourself in a trance. It is imperative to concentrate during this whole timeframe.

Stage 2

Set weight reduction objectives for yourself. Focus on a precise number of pounds you need to lose and a particular time you need to lose it. Examine this objective out loud before you start.

Stage 3

Close your eyes, and relax your body until it is totally limp. Focus on this profound relaxation for 3 minutes until you feel a warm sensation from your skull to your feet. After the sensation is felt, loosen up that piece of your body. You will be in a trance state.

Stage 4

Envision your optimal self in a relaxed state. Consider how you will see the world, how others will see you, and how great it will feel to be solid and fit as a fiddle. Take a good look at your body in its fit, trim state.

Stage 5

Return to your current state gradually. Be certain you bring the feelings of the inner experience back with you. Doing this day by day will prepare your brain to feel how great it will be to shed pounds. You will, step by step, build the mechanisms important to get in shape.

Self-Hypnosis: How Do We Do It?

Self-hypnosis follows the rules and techniques of classic hypnosis, with the difference that the hypnotherapist is yourself.

The Preparation

It is recommended to practice self-hypnosis while sitting on a comfortable armchair or sofa, feet flat on the floor, and hands on your thighs. All in complete silence, of course: you need to turn off your laptop, phone, and the TV!

Then we close our eyes and create a vacuum. This moment is close to meditation: it is a matter of becoming aware of each part of your body, starting from the feet and gradually going up to the head, breathing deeply.

It is only once completely relaxed that we can begin the autosuggestion phase.

Autosuggestion

The first rule of self-hypnosis (and hypnosis) is to treat only one problem at a time. If you suffer from both anxiety and lack of self-confidence, you devote a separate session to each of these problems.

Once the problem has been identified, we mentally address the unconscious to guide it toward resolving this problem.

This is where rule number 2 comes in: self-hypnosis is autosuggestion. It should not be a set of self-imposed orders. Sentences must always be positive. For example, we don't say, "you shouldn't be afraid," but "I'm not afraid anymore."

Also, we favor positive terms: better to say, "I know I will succeed" rather than "I no longer know failure" because failure is a strong and negative word on which the unconscious can focus.

Visualization

The secret to an effective self-hypnosis session, like hypnosis, is visualization.

It is a question of imagining oneself in precise situations and of printing images in the unconscious.

For example, to deal with the lack of self-confidence in a period of unemployment and with a goal to possible job interviews, it can be useful to imagine yourself working in a company (a more positive situation than a research job), for example, giving a presentation at a meeting with poise, and being applauded by his collaborators.

If the words guide the unconscious, the images mark it much more deeply.

Managing your emotions is very important when you want to lose weight.

Some hypnotists, still too few, know how to induce a hypnotic trance deep enough to be able to establish motivation, love, self-esteem, indifference, disgust, stomach constriction, and many other hypnosis techniques, which over time, allow their clients to lose weight.

A session of hypnosis, like a session of self-hypnosis, must be imagined in three acts: induction, which aims at physical relaxation and sensory isolation, followed by a rapid stage, almost brutal, when the act of hypnosis becomes a sort of spectacle, which aims at intellectual concentration and to make it clear to your brain that it is a transition from a state of consciousness towards an exterior state of consciousness. Then it turns towards the inside and finally to the hypnotic trance itself.

Your hypnosis practitioner can help with sleep disorders, anxiety, sexual disorders, addictions, food compulsions, eating disorders (bulimia, anorexia), mania, stuttering, migraines, ailments back, allergies, and weight loss. Therapeutic hypnosis can remedy many things, and this, sometimes, in very short times.

Hypnosis can plant the idea that you look forward to exercising your body. Soon, time at the gym will be the best part of your day. It may even become your favorite pastime!

Hypnosis, when properly implemented, is a valuable tool. There are millions of documented success stories of people overcoming problems with hypnosis. In addition to the weight problems discussed above, hypnosis can also help in other different areas.

Techniques of Weight Loss with Self-Hypnosis

Compassionate Self-Talk and Weight Loss

Poor self-talk is a negative attitude that has been strengthened over the decades, but it can be modified. Our minds are biochemical organs, so emotions arise mostly out of biology. Your thoughts don't define you. But they impact your behaviors. Recognize that your first line of thinking is always based on genetics; it is our inherent negative orientation, and if you don't like it, you should discard the first thinking.

This ensures you can choose whether or not you are choosing a different thought. Shunning your negative first thought and choosing to have a second thought is an important device that encourages you to pick the new, healthier thoughts and see yourself more favorably.

Critical self-talk is a common way in which our minds put issues first. It originates from a biological mechanism known as *Negativity Bias*.

Negativity bias is one of the factors that helped mankind survive in human history. It is the potential of our minds to rely on the bad for protection.

Take a minute to reflect on what type of stuff your inner voice is communicating to you right now, whenever you feel tempted to overeat or when you've consumed everything that you label as "bad." It's not really helpful, more often than not. Maybe you're admonishing yourself for consuming food you believe you're 'not supposed to have,' or maybe you're telling yourself labels or reminding yourself you're disappointed by your actions or wondering what certain people think about you and you ask yourself, "what's wrong with me?" Picture how you'd like it if other individuals were referring to you in the way you're talking to yourself. Imagine telling somebody you value these things. How does that leave you feeling? Probably you would not be pleased. Yet frequently deceiving yourself will lead to self-hatred, and the persistent inner battle between guilt and compensation is frustrating.

It's a cycle of finding consolation and then criticizing oneself, and it's mentally draining. Avoid allowing verbal abuse of yourself. You wouldn't accept it from somebody else, so turn the voice inside into something that supports you, embraces you, and is good; because you deserve it.

Applaud yourself for making the initial steps in permanently improving your life and admire all the commendable things you are achieving for yourself and everyone.

Self-compassion in self-critical people was also found to be important in enhancing weight reduction and addressing unhealthy eating behaviors. Psychologists believe that we've had it all backward. The simplest approach to shedding weight and feeling your best is to quit yo-yo dieting and continue by accepting who and what you are." Self-compassion is an infantile, gentler, more successful way to lose weight than starvation accompanied by self-loathing when you don't adhere to your food schedule. To certain individuals who have little to no empathy towards themselves, the 'positivity diet' method fits well, encouraging self-acceptance, committing to healthier food, and creating sustainable good lifestyle shifts towards a better self.

People usually always say bad things to themselves. Being harsh on oneself is not a means of shedding weight. Dieters who pass judgments on themselves all day, telling themselves mean words like: "I am huge. I'm out of shape" are setting themselves up to overeat. Healthy weight management simply has four components. One of them is self-compassion, and it binds all of the foundations together.

The three areas are compassion toward oneself, conscientious eating, self-hypnosis (imagining), and social assistance.

Self-compassion starts by flipping your inner critic around and getting a positive attitude to your mind when you've already made a less-than-perfect choice of food or succumbed to disordered eating patterns. It helps to note that it's a road to get a grip on eating problems, not the step many dieters are willing to take. Research has found that only a small dose of self-compassion will reduce harmful self-criticism and unpleasant emotions that can trigger mindless eating.

If you find that you're giving yourself a punishment with respect to your size or shape, focus on thinking kind thoughts. Instead of thinking "I cannot drop weight" or labeling yourself "big," "ugly," and other negative titles, remind yourself what you would say to a true friend: "Nobody is completely perfect." When you quit reaching for excellence and start loving you as you are, losing fat with a healthy, balanced eating plan is just normal.

Do some self-hypnosis or relaxing meditation to banish self-hatred. Self-hypnosis basically guides your awareness, intensifies your breathing, and then expands your mind to fresh thoughts and experiences. You should motivate yourself with positive thoughts that appeal to you, like, "I want more and more healthy and good food."

Or, "I love the organic flavor of healthy grains every day and in every way." Choose something that is inspiring and valuable to you. Offer a suggestion to yourself, then practice with a calm and concentrated mind.

Self-hypnosis is an appropriate solution to shift from harmful diets, which are less than ideal, and to alter the attitudes you have for food. As we concentrate on healthier food and weight reduction targets, intentionally and subconsciously, this continuous awareness is our friend in implementing positive habits and activities that promote a fulfilled life.

The benefits of self-compassion relative to conventional weight loss regimens are that it is more about creating progress internally that can promote a healthy lifestyle on a permanent basis. A self-loathing individual is unable to make better everyday food decisions. Understanding different ways to think of you and feel for yourself is supposed to develop better and healthier patterns. Most workout programs and other weight-loss strategies revolve around the deprivation and abuse that stimulate unpleasant emotions. You stay on the self-hate approach. You continue taking the small portions no matter how starved you are. When you feel tired, you keep ongoing. "No gain without suffering" becomes your mantra.

While you're on vacation, you keep tracking portions, sugar and feel ashamed if you screw up.

So, when you're traveling, you stuff your suitcase with all your diet snacks. It is not positive, and it is not nice. Alternatively, seek and approach yourself with plenty of self-love. You'll be more willing to eat while you're starving and quit when you're finished, relax when you're exhausted, and walk while you're feeling energized. So, as you do this, you will automatically lose weight.

Self-Compassionate Exercise

1. Jot down a summary of all the good stuff about yourself in your notebook. For instance: "I'm a good friend and have time to listen to others" or "I show patience with my family" or "I take great care of my dogs" and "I'm a genuine person."

2. Accept all the positive stuff you have and then know that you accept that you need to improve your food choices and that you are moving towards a better, safer life.

3. Show empathy and consideration through your internal monologue whenever you believe you've gotten off course, just as you would if a kid made an error or got lost. Your internal monologue should be positive and compassionate; it's a part of you, after all, and every part of your efforts for your well-being.

Autosuggestion Under Self-Hypnosis

By now, you have understood the power of self-talk for weight loss. Now, we're going to elaborate on how you can use the concept of positive self-talk to make hypnotic autosuggestions for weight loss.

They say, "You become whatever you tell yourself." Autosuggestion operates around the premise that first, we have to modify our thought in order to alter our habits, characteristics, or behaviors. Autosuggestion includes regularly stocking up the subconscious mind with constructive guidance. Your subconscious mind absorbs knowledge from the senses endlessly; however, most of it is negative. Your rational mind is operating on the knowledge the subconscious mind lets in. One approach to do that is by utilizing affirmations, which are optimistic words that you say every day on a daily basis, usually as you awaken and before bed. Such comments apply to everything you want to accomplish. In order to work with autosuggestion, you have to clear your head of any unpleasant thinking as quickly as it surfaces.

Training the subconscious mind with autosuggestion is a mental training technique created by each person that encourages the subconscious mind to embrace constructive thoughts and expectations, and from these exercises, its latent power in achieving those goals.

With the following methods, you'll already be well on your path to teaching the subconscious mind with autosuggestion.

The autosuggestion is focused on the principle of reinforcement. The continuous repetition of positive thinking is utilized to establish targets, which creates a clear link between the rational and the subconscious mind, enabling the subconscious mind to influence the conscious mind. Through this cycle of reinforcement of encouraging affirmations, the subconscious is ready to experience the right path to achieve the goal.

Weight Loss Affirmations

- "I'm able to shed fat now."
- I embrace the shape of my body and recognize the beauty it contains.
- "I deserve perfect well-being now, and I embrace it."

- "I let go of associations that aren't for my higher purpose anymore."
- "I am letting go of undesirable behavior surrounding food."
- "I feel comfortable with my body."
- "I can turn my healthy practices into a balanced lifestyle."
- "I trust in my capacity to value myself genuinely for who I am."
- "I am the creator of my destiny."
- "I'm empowering myself to make better judgments and choices."
- "I am compassionate with myself and others."
- "I love to move my body every day."
- "I feel confident."
- "I'm letting go of any remorse that I carry over food decisions."
- "Health and slimming are easy to achieve for me."
- "I have faith and confidence in the future."
- "I listen to everything my body demands of me."
- "I eat what I like, and when I begin to feel satisfied, I stop."
- "I love my meals, and I eat thoughtfully."
- "I keep moving closer to my healthy weight every day."
- "I am fortunate for the body that I inhabit and for all that it does for me."
- "I listen lovingly to what my body wants."
- "I feed myself with fresh fruit and vegetables and with water."
- "I work out every day."
- "I feed more attentively, and I savor every morsel."
- "I have the skills needed to hit my target weight."
- "I make deliberate choices that help me attain my target weight."
- "Nutrition and weight loss are the highest priority for me."
- "I work on my attitude daily so that I feel positive."
- "I am getting slimmer, happier, and fitter every day."
- "I love and support all parts of myself."
- "I love and respect every aspect of my body."
- "Staying active and lean each day is simpler for me."

TIPS FOR SUCCESSFUL AUTOSUGGESTIONS

1. **Use it in the Present Tense.** The subconscious domain just doesn't know about time—the time is frozen, so all information is received as though it were occurring right now. State your suggestions in the present. Otherwise, the result you desire would only be in the future, waiting to occur. So instead of saying, "I'm going to walk daily," it will be a more powerful expression as, "I enjoy walking daily!"

2. **When you use the present tense, you ought to be clear on where, when, how, and so on.** Using phrases like "I am" or "I believe" is more successful than "I will." It even may be detrimental to your weight loss goals. Avoid making suggestions that include not doing something that you intend to alter any further. Rather, concentrate on words and resulting visualization of the necessary behavioral and mindset improvements that will help the goals.

   Suggestions are often more helpful when considering what you want to achieve rather than what you run away from. "I'm relaxed" is stronger than "I'm not nervous," for starters. "I'm going to stop overeating with ease" is better than "I'm going to try and quit overeating," as the term "try" suggests effort and challenge. The thoughts are best worded in the present, as though they are occurring right now.

3. **Activate the Suggestion.** Not only do you want the terms that indicate behavior, performing, and acting, but you want them to include a course of action. That may be a suggestion to behave attentively, stroll after supper, take a glass of water in the morning, etc.

4. **Add your own name.** Obviously, when you speak to yourself, you listen more! Make constructive feedback that applauds you for doing good, say, "Hey Michael, I admire the way you always do XYZ!" What a fantastic antidote to years of destructive self-hatred. Everyone should add a positive suggestion in their life.

5. **Keep it short.** The portion of the mind that you want to touch is still pretty infantile and takes information literally. You don't need complex words here, so avoid complicated, scientific, or philosophical terminology.

6. **Say it as you believe it.** Hypnotic instructions are delivered in quiet. However, you have to reiterate the ideas as though you believe what you say.

7. **Repeat your suggestions.** Repeat your suggestions. Repeating your suggestions is one of the most significant principles when doing self-hypnosis.

8. **Personalize it.** Until someone admits and acknowledges that no one will convince them to do it, they cannot develop ownership for anything. Personal responsibility is needed to make lasting lifestyle adjustments to let go of guilt or reliance on others. Perhaps some would change because of their own suggestions, while several people still consider themselves helpless.

9. **In time, you will realize that listening to your speech repeating the ideas is more than enough.** Therefore, worrying critically about constructive thoughts would be less necessary.

Stages of Self-Hypnosis

Diving into your considerations and thoughts is that delicate excursion into the focal point of yourself called "going into a stupor." The straightforward methods of self-hypnosis incorporate going into a daze, deepening the daze, utilizing that daze state to give messages and recommendations to the mind-body, and coming out of the daze.

SUBCONSCIOUS MIND (OR UNCONSCIOUS MIND)

This is the bit of our mind that performs capacities and procedures beneath our reasoning mindfulness.

It is the mind of the body. It inhales us, digests, makes our hearts beat, and as a rule, deals with our automatic physical procedures for us.

It can likewise instruct us to pick a bit of new mango rather than chocolate cake, to quit eating when we are full, or to appreciate a stroll in the recreation center.

GOING INTO TRANCE

When you are utilizing the stupor at this point, take notice of the sound. I will be your guide as you go into a daze. I will utilize a daze enlistment strategy that you will discover quieting and centering. You have most likely observed the swinging watch technique in motion pictures, which is thirty-five years of training I have never observed anybody use. Yet, there is a vast number of approaches to concentrate on going into a stupor. You may gaze at a spot on the divider, utilize a breathing procedure, or use dynamic body unwinding. You will hear an assortment of acceptance strategies on the stupor sound. They are just the prompts or the signs that you are providing for yourself to state, "I am going into a daze" or "I will do my hypnosis currently." Going into a trance can likewise be thought of as "letting yourself dream... intentionally."

You are letting yourself become consumed in your contemplations and thoughts, exceptionally invested, and permitting yourself to imagine or envision what you want as accomplished and genuine. There is no "going under." Instead, there is a beautiful encounter of going inside.

COGNIZANT MIND

This is the "thinking mind" or the piece of the mind that gives us our mindfulness or feeling of knowing and oversees our deliberate capacities. For instance, our cognizant mind takes that second bit of pie at the meal, swipes the check card at the market, and moves the fork to our mouth.

Different Methods of Self-Hypnosis

THE BETTY ERICKSON METHOD

Here I'll summarize the most practical points of the method of Betty Erickson, wife of Milton Erickson, the most famous hypnotist of 1900.

Choose something you don't like about yourself. Turn it into an image, and then turn this image into a positive one. If you don't like your body shape, take a picture of your body, then turn it into an image of your beautiful self with a body you would like to have.

Before inducing self-hypnosis, give yourself a time limit before hypnotizing yourself mentally or better yet, saying aloud the following sentence, "I induce self-hypnosis for X minutes." Your mind will keep time like a Swiss watch.

How Do You Practice?

Take three objects around you, preferably small and bright, like a door handle, a light spot on a painting, etc., and fix your attention on each one of them. Take three sounds from your environment, traffic, fridge noise, etc., and fix your attention on each one. Take three sensations you are feeling, the itchy nose, tingling in the leg, the feeling of air passing through the nose, etc. It's better to focus on unusual sensations, to which attention is not usually drawn, such as the sensation of the right foot inside the shoe. Don't fix your attention for too long, just enough to make you aware of what you are seeing, feeling, or trying. The mind is quick. Then, in the same way, switch to two objects, two sounds, two sensations. Always be calm while switching to an object, a sound, a sensation. If you have perfectly done things, you are in a trance, ready for the next step.

Now let your mind wander, as you did in class when the teacher spoke and you looked out of the window, and you were in another place, in another time, in another space, in a place where you would have liked to be, so completely forget about everything else. Now recall the initial image. Perhaps the mind wanders; from time to time, it gets distracted, maybe it goes adrift, but it doesn't matter. As soon as you can, take the initial image, and start working on it. Do not make efforts to try to remind you of what it means or what it is. Your mind works according to mental associations; let it work at its best without unnecessarily disturbing it: it knows what it must do. Manipulate the image, play with it a little.

See if it looks brighter, or if it is smaller, or it is more pleasant. If it is a moving image, send it back and forth in slow motion or speed it up. If the initial image always gets worse, replace it instantly with the second image.

Reorientation, also known as awakening, marks the end of self-hypnotic induction. Enjoy your new image, savor it as much as you like, and when you have done this, open your eyes. If you are unable to give yourself enough time, set limits before entering self-hypnosis. When you are satisfied with the work done, count quietly to yourself from one to ten and wake up and open your eyes.

THE BENSON METHOD

Herbert Benson, in his famous book titled 'Relaxation Response,' describes the methods and results of some tests carried out on a group of meditators dedicated to "transcendental meditation" to reach concentration. Benson suggested a method of relaxation based on the concentration of the mind on a single idea, which was incorporated in the Eastern disciplines. The technique includes the following steps:

- Meditate on one word, but you can choose an object or something else if you want to.
- Now, it's time to sit down in a quiet place and close your eyes. Relax the muscles and direct attention to the breath.
- Think silently about the object of meditation and continue to do so for 10–20 minutes. If you find that you have lost the object of meditation, gather your focus again on the original object.
- Once the set time is reached, open your eyes and stretch yourself well for some additional minutes. Obviously, to perform better, you will need to practice.

Benson proposes this exercise as a meditation practice.

In reality, there are no differences between the hypnotic state and that achieved with meditation. This is one of the most straightforward self-hypnosis exercises you can do.

Here is another simple technique that was developed by the first hypnotists because it leads to a satisfactory state of trance in a reasonable time. It can be used to enter self-hypnosis in a short time.

Now, it's time to sit down in a quiet place and close your eyes. Relax the muscles and direct attention to the breath.

Begin to open and close your eyes by counting slowly. Open your eyes at the odd numbers close them at the even numbers. Continue counting very slowly and slowing down the numbering of even numbers.

After a few numbers, your eyes become tired, and you find it difficult to open them at odd numbers.

Continue counting while you can open your eyes at the odd numbers. If you cannot do it, it means you are in a trance.

Go deeper by slowly counting twenty other numbers. Let yourself go to the images, to the sensations, and to the words that come to mind. To wake up from the trance, count from one to five, and open your eyes at five.

These are examples of techniques, but no one is preventing you from devising others, as long as the underlying assumption is maintained: concentration on a single idea.

We, as a whole, essentially need time to unwind, to dream, to imagine.

It is refreshing to the physical body and restoring to the soul. At the point when we practice our hypnosis, it offers us simply that: an exceptionally close to home time to animate and enhance our mind and body. The training is done essentially. You don't require anything over an agreeable and safe spot.

How to Enhance Self-Hypnosis Experience
KNOW IF YOUR SELF-HYPNOSIS IS WORKING

There are some small things you can do physically to know if hypnosis is really working for you, especially if you are a self-hypnosis beginner.

Put both your hands together, palm-to-palm tightly and keep them in this position throughout your hypnotic state. Imagine your hands superglued together and keep saying, "My hands can't come apart. They are stuck together."

Now try to pull them apart. If you are not able to do so, then you're in the right state of hypnosis.

Another method to test the effectiveness of your self-hypnosis is to concentrate on how heavy one of your arms is becoming and if it is getting heavier and heavier throughout your session. Imagine a heavy-weight is placed on your arm, which is making it difficult to lift your arm.

Now try to raise that arm up into the air. If you are failing at doing this, then you are in the right hypnosis state.

WHAT TO DO IF SELF-HYPNOSIS DOESN'T WORK

Have you ever encountered the annoyance of having a name on the tip of your tongue? The more you try to recall the name, the more difficult it gets to remember. And then, when you relax, the name automatically comes back to you.

Mistakes That People Make Often

Learning self-hypnosis is not that hard, but it is easy for newbies to make mistakes. However, try to avoid making the following beginner mistakes when you begin learning self-hypnosis, and you'll be off to a great start:

EXPECTING TOO MUCH

Many people regard self-hypnosis as a miracle cure and thus become disappointed if they don't get the desired result in their very first attempt. Never expect to achieve your goal with just one or two sessions, especially if you are a newbie. You need to allow it to take time in order to be effective.

FAILURE TO RELAX ENOUGH

You are required to quieten your body and mind to maintain a hypnotic state. Regular meditation will assist you in learning the focus that you will need in order to utilize self-hypnosis effectively.

FAILURE OF BEING OPEN TO THE SELF-HYPNOSIS EXPERIENCE

You'll need to work through any psychological blocks you have about hypnosis before doing a hypnotic session.

FAILURE TO PREPARE ENOUGH AHEAD OF TIME

Hypnotherapy takes time and preparation to use as an effective therapeutic tool. Keep in mind that, like any other skill, self-hypnosis needs to be learned and practiced before you can perform it well and obtain your desired benefits.

Tips to Manifest Your Best Through Self-Hypnosis

KEEP YOURSELF HYDRATED

Drink water before the session to ensure that you are hydrated since being hydrated is helpful in any practice of negative energy clearing.

BE RELAXED

Relaxation is an important element of self-hypnosis since when you relax the mind and body, you clear the way for an opportunity to welcome effective life changing changes. Although self-hypnosis is constructed to provide you with relaxation, you can further enhance the experience by getting rid of your tension and stress by having a home massage or a relaxing bath or doing some form of exercise.

AVOID STRUGGLING WITH YOUR EMOTIONS

As a newbie, it can be frustrating and difficult to obtain a peaceful mind state. Clearing your mind may induce the flow of different kinds of emotions and make you unstable. Try to overlook these emotions and concentrate more on finding peace in your mind.

The last and essential thing you must know to enhance your hypnotic experience is that it's ok if you're unable to achieve. The world won't come to a standstill, the sun won't stop rising; neither will the sky come falling if you're not able to obtain your goals. Success and failure both are cyclic in nature and are a part of our life.

Thus, don't get obsessed with goals, rather be passionate about them. Work towards it, never end up spending more time worrying about it. Sooner or later, you'll surely be the winner.

5

Self-Hypnosis for Self Improvement

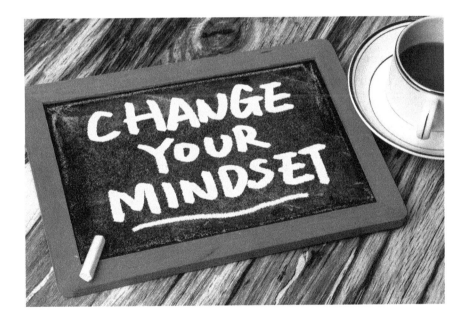

You control the crucial elements that make self-hypnosis work for you. Actually, these elements, which might be motivation, belief, and expectation, are the equal components that create your enjoyment of fulfillment for any aim you choose. Let us look at each element and how you may use it to carry out your hypnosis.

How to Love Your Body?

Among the motives why we communicate a lot about loving yourself is because that is where your healthy self-popularity has to begin. If you do not love yourself now, even having the attractive looks of a Paul Newman or a Marilyn Monroe cannot deliver that to you. By the way, did you recognize that Marilyn Monroe wore a size 14?

Stand in front of a mirror and examine your body. Begin with your head and work down through each part of your body. Recall some things this body element has achieved for you.

Tell it "thank you" for something specific that it did for you.

Continue to the next body part.

After accomplishing your feet and toes, go back to your head. Proceed down your frame, telling each body component,

"I love you."

I can assure you that you are on your way to achieving your dream weight.

MOTIVATION

Motivation is the electricity for your choice of what you want. Wanting is a feeling that you may control. For most of your life, you have managed your preference or worked through limiting it or denying it. You may be superb at controlling your goals and needs in some regions and susceptible or unpracticed in others.

Since this is a "diet" book, you could have already told yourself to listen that this "diet" will be just like the others that have informed you that you must deny yourself or limit. The alternative diets of the past have instructed you what no longer need, and the emphasis may also have been on "no longer trying" foods that you have grown to love. Welcome to a fresh way of treating yourself; we can inspire you to get even higher at "looking." We do not cover denial in this guide.

Your motivation is a key factor and one of the fundamental substances.

We want you to focus your strength of looking not closer to food but closer to the incentive that truly tells your mind-body what you want it to create: best weight. We inspire you to get into the reality of wanting your perfect weight. Here is an example. Let's say you are in a swimming pool, and abruptly you breathe in a mouthful of water.

At that moment, you need one element, a breath of air. It feels like life or death, and a breath of air is the handiest factor on your mind at that moment. The looking is so severe and powerful that it overshadows all other thoughts and propels you to do anything it takes to get that breath of air. That is how much we need you to crave the weight and body image you seek.

BELIEF AND BELIEVING

Beliefs are the thoughts valid to you. They don't need to be scientifically proven to be real for you. If you are aware of it or not, your movements, both conscious and subconscious, are functions of your beliefs. Even though your ideas are within the form of mind and thoughts, they shape your experience by affecting your moves in life.

If you trust that animals make proper companions, you probably have a cat or dog or parrot or a ferret or two. If you agree that coffee will keep you up at night, you probably no longer drink espresso before going to bed.

Remember your make-accept some of these beliefs as true since you were a child.

Your capacity to fabricate a belief is just as sturdy now as while you were young. It can be a touch rusty, and you may want a bit of practice; however, while you allow yourself to fake and let yourself believe in what you're pretending, you will find out a powerful tool. You will discover that this is a wonderfully effective way to deliver your intentions, the ones with messages of what you need, to all the cells and tissues and organs of your body, which reply by bringing that purpose into reality for you.

We can't say this enough: thoughts are things. The thoughts, the pictures, the words you put in your mind emerge as the messages your self-hypnosis conveys to your mind-body, turning your ideal body into truth. Pretending is choosing what to consider and turning it into ideas you can absorb. Just as a magnifying glass can create rays of sunlight, you can raise the awareness of your mental power to make your thoughts and ideas ideal for your shape.

EXPECTATION

You might not continually get what you need; however, you can get what you expect. Expectations incorporate the energy of beliefs and grow to be the outcomes of what's believed. Here is an example of a way to "expect." When you sat down to examine this book, you did not observe the chair or sofa to check its capability to maintain your weight.

You just sat down without thinking about it. You did not have to consider it because a part of you is confident, and has a lot of faith in the chair, that you just "expected" it to support you.

That is a way to expect a suitable bodyweight you desire. Keeping this in your thoughts, consider what you are saying to yourself and others concerning your frame and weight expectations. "I continually gain weight over the holidays." "Last night, I ate two portions of cake, and this morning I am two pounds heavier."

MIND-BODY IN FOCUS

Each of the essential elements can produce powerful consequences whilst focused inside the thoughts-frame. However, when these elements align properly in the process of self-hypnosis, their effectiveness is magnified a hundredfold. Self-hypnosis is a way of developing your desires.

You might suppose this sounds magical or too exact to be true; however, that is relative to what you've experienced so far in your life.

These ideas can be very new to you. Here is an example of the "relative" nature of recent thoughts. Imagine someone gives you a personal jet that is beautifully designed with costly appointments and a well-educated crew. It is an amazing gift, and you get to reveal this engineering marvel to some individuals who have never seen anything like it.

Let us say that your pilot flies you back in time to just before December 17, 1903, whilst the Wright brothers introduced their first flight at Kitty Hawk.

You are eager to reveal this wonder of engineering to the Wright brothers, who come to greet you. What might happen? Perhaps they will be scared and won't trust that it's possible to fly for in a metal bird. You could offer them a ride, and they might run from you. People can reject new thoughts, even when they're good.

The philosopher Arthur Schopenhauer said, "Every man takes the limits of his own field of vision for the limits of the world." Stretch your world view and allow yourself the opportunity to end up acquainted with the thoughts of self-hypnosis.

In this guide, we are offering you thoughts that could stretch your creativeness and reduce your clothing size. To say that self-hypnosis is a process through which you create your reality may also seem too exact to be proper or even unbelievable, perhaps as outstanding as a time system is for some. That is fine right now, but open your mind and creativeness to the opportunities that this offers you to get your ideal body weight. Let your self-trust that this procedure is actual and authentic because it's far, and because it is predicated upon your notion to end up true.

Your subconscious (mind-body) uses the mixture of what you want (motivation), what you accept as true, and what you count on as a blueprint for action.

You carry the effects by using your thoughts-frame (subconsciously) and not by questioning or analyzing.

If someone touches an icy floor that she believes could be hot, she can produce a blister or burn response. Conversely, someone that touches a hot surface that doesn't think that it is cool may not produce a burn response. People who stroll over hot coals while imagining that they're cool may also enjoy a thermal injury (some minor sizzling on the soles of their feet); however, their immune system does not respond with a burn (blistering, pain, etc.) because their minds inform our bodies how to react.

Again, it's the alignment of all three of the important substances that make this workable:

- Seek to do it
- Believe it's doable
- Watching for success

These are the keys to fulfillment. Your body carries your ideas. Your beliefs direct your actions, which form your experience.

Some describe this method as growing your success or developing your experience in life. In our culture, we see this described inside the motivational and wonderful mental attitude literature. We can see it in many areas of metaphysics. You also can look back to the ancients and notice it described in the phrases of the ancient period.

In the present age of integrative medicine and psychology, we name it self-hypnosis or mind-body remedy. There are now several scientific studies that show amazing results for impulse control, wound healing, bodily alteration, and lots more healthy benefits than we previously thought possible.

Beliefs and How They Affect Weight Loss

Does your conviction hold you back? There are several schools of thinking regarding a belief. But ultimately, a belief is what we really "think" or "learn." The negative side of a belief is that our life experiences shape all our values, from childhood onwards. Some of us heard derogatory comments from those around us when we grew up, and people might have said stuff like 'you've just got big bones' or 'being overweight runs in your family' We may have believed some of them, even without realizing it. A conviction is not simply about 'knowing' to be true. We can 'think' and make it a belief.

The meaning of "belief" is somewhat hazy. Beliefs are learned but can be mixed with our own hands. This is one reason the word belief has so many schools of thought.

CHOOSING YOUR BELIEFS

You can pick your beliefs. You can also pick what to believe and what you see within the experience of "See it to consider it" or "Seeing is believing." This is very easy to do.

You revel in something together with your senses, and that could be a familiar way of choosing whether it is plausible or not. But you could also choose to consider it first after which you see it, which also requires a few exercises.

Most people find it less complicated to let the world tell them what is actual or what to agree with. The television, media, newspapers, books, teachers, and professionals bombard us with what to believe. You grew up learning about the world and yourself from many external sources.

This brought about an acquainted pattern of looking at and receiving data about the world from people other than yourself, and you chose which information to make a part of your belief system. This included beliefs about your body. For example, while your belly makes a rumbling sound, you trust that means you are hungry. Or you sense that you are nauseous and trust you are sick. Both are examples of found events: you discovered a connection once and believed it.

With this in mind, which of these statements would help you experience the perfect weight you desire: "I just look at food and gain weight" or "I can eat whatever and my weight remains the same" Surely the latter. But which statement do you personally believe to be proper for you? Again, it will probably have been passed to you together with your notion.

We will assist you with the thoughts, language, and photographs that plan effective hypnotic pointers; however, you have got total control over what you pick to believe.

As you examine the thoughts in this e-book, you'll make many choices for yourself. We wholeheartedly inspire you to choose to accept them as true, so you can see them for yourself. Your unconscious (thoughts-frame) cannot identify the difference and can act on what you pick either way. Why choose what you no longer need?

The Energy of Emotions

Not all minds and ideas show themselves to you. Only those that have the strength of their feelings, with perception and expectation that something will happen, manifest themselves. Your feelings or emotions are a shape of energy that affects this system of creation. If you have a strong feeling or a perception, it contains strength. That strength creates joy and similarly reinforces your beliefs and expectations. We are talking about the combined energy of your thoughts, your beliefs, your expectancies, and what you need. The mental energy behind what you want and what you let yourself need creates motivation. So perhaps you could see that it is vital to let yourself truly want something with top-rate feelings. If you combine feeling with need, you empower the manner in which you are placing these into motion within you.

Make sure that your feelings remain nice. You can determine when they are fine or poor by how they make you feel.

It's simple. Emotions that make you feel excellent are helpful, and feelings that make you feel awful are terrible. Keep all of those energies nice by focusing on desires, beliefs, and expectations. If you have terrible feelings in mind, they will damage your motivation.

If you have got a fine mind and emotions, they will reinforce your motivation. Thoughts, ideas, and expectations are equal-possibility energies. You can attract them and produce high quality or terrible results and outcomes. If you are bad, assume poor results. If you are superb, expect fantastic results. In this way, any thought, belief, or expectation produces a bad or high-quality result. It's a straightforward decision—if you need success, seek tremendous energy from a tremendous mind and feelings.

Choosing Your Feelings

Your mind/body also perceives your notion based on your underlying feeling. Here is an example. Let us say you need to consider something that will help you achieve your goal. You compose an affirmation and begin announcing it aloud to yourself. Affirmations are an incredible way to create fantastic ideas. Saying the affirmations allows your ears to pay attention, and your voice communicates them.

This, too, is a way of choosing your ideas and reinforcing them. For example, you can say the confirmation, "I am lighter and thinner today." But what do you experience? If you "experience" you are overweight or feel that the confirmation is untrue and tell yourself the confirmation anyway, there may be a conflict.

What you feel is another way that your unconscious perceives your belief or what you keep as genuine. It is vital that your feelings are in alignment with your affirmations and your desires, beliefs, and expectations. Remember, emotions are power. You can ask, "But what if I don't agree with what I am telling myself?" Do it anyway. It is better than focusing the strength of your feelings, desires, and beliefs on a poor route. It is also a step inside the path you need to proceed.

Is It All in Your Mind?

Now you'll be thinking maybe the ideas you are studying about self-hypnosis are "all on your mind." That is a truthful question. It changed into the normal notion that hypnosis became a psychological tool that is most effective at involving the mind.

However, studies show that it involves each part of the body and mind. A report inside the American Journal of Psychiatry in 2000 used PET brain scans to examine the regions of the mind activated by shade and gray sunglasses.

They found that after the proven result of hypnotized topics, the gray color had changed into shade, the elements of the mind that the method color activated, and the gray-color processing areas were not.

And whilst they proved the shade pattern once instructed, it became a gray color. The best regions of the mind that nature had activated in the procedure were gray shades.

Research in Neuro-Image in 2004 used useful MRI mind scanning to look at the parts of the mind activated by using pain. Subjects were given hypnotic pointers to be in pain. The researchers found that hypnotically produced pain and physically produced ache activated the same components of the brain.

What these studies tell us is, "Yes, it's far in your mind... and your body." Your body responds to ideas, thoughts, expectations, and hypnotic hints as real totally and physically.

How Do You Want Your Frame to Respond?

Remember, you cannot make any mistakes with this guide. You could make no mistakes to your achievement of weight loss. If any unwanted effects occur, you honestly just change or adjust some things. You might adjust what you want or believe, or what you expect, or you might alternate your feelings.

If you don't like the results, change what you're doing. You can change what is causing the consequences until the effects are steady with what you want to have happened.

Whenever you are aware of unwanted results, you could map out an alternative route for where you need to go. Your new map comprises what you need, believe, and expect, with a sense of gratitude, and consider that it's guaranteed.

No longer waste time or power even considering what you do not want. Even worse than that is losing your power on what you might think of as obstacles or resistance to your success. Merely questioning these directions gives power to them. Focus your brain and mental energy on the outcomes you want to enjoy. Thoughts, ideas, and expectancies are energy. Use your energy wisely. Direct all the strength should to your superb results.

Belief Never Fails... Even When False

Belief does not fail, ever. Your ideas and expectations will never fail you. They will always prove themselves true, even when they're false beliefs. In 2005, Dr. Elizabeth Loftus supplied the effects of a study on false beliefs to the National Academy of Science. She created a false memory (something untrue) on a particular food once made the study subjects sick when they were children.

The outcomes confirmed that the individuals later averted consuming those meals, which changed into presenting the notion as true. Are you acting out something as true? Examine if it's far from a belief that benefits you.

Fighting Anxiety and Stress

Stress and anxiety are the all-natural reactions of the body to tension. It is a feeling of concern or fear concerning what is ahead. Activities such as giving a speech, going for a work interview, or the very first day of college may create most of the individuals to feel scared or worried.

Most of us have nervous feelings at some point in our lives. Feeling terrified or stressed is a typical response to demanding as well as hazardous circumstances. We can feel tense as well as nervous before a presentation, doing exams at universities, or beginning a new job.

Typically, once we have found out how to conquer a frustrating circumstance, our anxiety, then our fears will cool down. At times, the anxious concerns can be with us after a problematic situation has passed.

Feelings of worry, distress, and fear can take over. We can feel down with anxiety signs, which can affect us for a very long time.

ANXIOUSNESS TEST

Anxiousness is hard to detect. Nonetheless, a medical anxiety diagnosis requires a lengthy process of psychological health and wellness analyses, mental surveys, and a medical examination.

Some doctors could do a physical examination, urine, or blood tests to eliminate significant clinical problems, which can add to indicators you are suffering from stress.

Different anxiousness ranges, and tests, are also used to help your medical professional to evaluate the degree of anxiety you are experiencing.

WHAT CAUSES ANXIETY

Most doctors do not completely recognize what creates anxiousness. It is thought that specific stressful experiences can trigger anxiousness in people who are prone to it. Genes could likewise play a vital role in stress and anxiety. In other instances, your stress and anxiety may be caused by a hidden health and wellness issue, which can be the very first indicator of mental disease.

ANXIETY THERAPY

You will uncover different treatment choices with your medical professional if you have been identified with anxiety.

For some people, medical treatment is not required. Lifestyle modifications may be adequate to deal with the signs.

In extreme cases, complementary therapy could help you conquer the symptoms and also can lead to you handling your anxiety.

Therapy for anxiety comes under two categories: medication and treatment. Sitting with a hypnotherapist or specialist might help you in understanding the devices to use as well as methods to handle your anxiety when the panic sets in.

Common anxiety medications offered are antidepressants. They work to stop episodes of anxiety, fend off the most serious indicators of the condition, and also balance mind chemistry.

Hypnosis is now being used as a fantastic treatment for people with panic attacks as well as a therapy for fears. It is ideal for people that can't or does not wish to use medication. It's an excellent therapy choice for those dealing with signs despite other interventions.

Research study has shown that hypnosis is also efficient at alleviating symptoms of widespread anxiety problems and even different types of stress and depression problems.

HELP AND TREATMENT

The hypnotherapist can help you to feel in control of your problems if you're seeking for the best assistance and also treatment.

Anxiety starts from worrying. In case of a generalized stress and anxiety attack, there are hidden lies in the subconscious mind.

Hypnosis puts your body in a state of relaxation in which it is possible to speak with your subconscious mind. That location is the part of the brain, which is responsible for automatic practices, ideas, and also sensations. When you are under hypnosis, the hypnotherapist can begin to alter the stressing thought patterns. This will change the fear, negative messages which contribute to the signs and symptoms of stress and anxiety.

Your hypnotherapist can give you ideas to bypass the adverse messages with affirming ones that support feelings of calmness and also relaxation.

Better, in contrast to medications, hypnosis is devoid of adverse effects.

6

Hypnosis for Weight Reduction

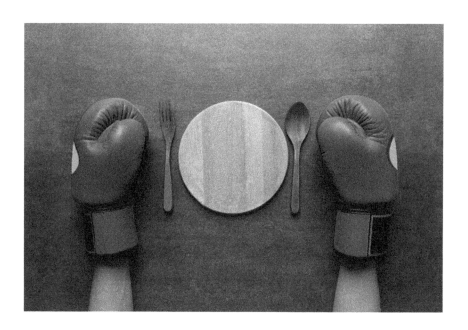

Hypnosis itself has been used for many different things, ranging from overcoming addictions or habits to helping people increase their sense of self-esteem and self-confidence. In some cases, people will even use hypnosis and guided visualization to relax their minds or take a small break from the stresses of their day-to-day lives. In many ways, these "mini-vacations" are similar to daydreaming, but they tend to be more structured and intentional.

How Does Hypnosis for Weight Loss Work?

Since they lead a sedentary way of life, this can be one factor why individuals are obese, but it is not. It's merely because they have a desire to consume more than "regular" people. When our bodies feel full, then we are supposed to stop wasting.

For obese individuals, when they feel full and are no longer starving, they continue to eat. For lots of obese people, this is one of the types of satisfaction that they can get.

Since it resets an individual's relationship with food, hypnosis is very useful.

Food is supposed to taste good; that's what kept us alive for thousands of years—the cravings to head out and get food to please the appetite with. When you are no longer starving, then you need to stop eating.

Hypnosis is not what many people think it is. Because of old movies and performers, many people tend to think that hypnosis is some form of party trick that results in people struggling to have any control over themselves and their behaviors. This is not at all true. When you engage in hypnosis, you always control yourself, your body, and your behaviors. The suggestions being offered to you in guided meditations, such as the ones you will follow in this book, are just that: suggestions. Because hypnosis is not the absolute power that many movies depict, it can take a few tries with hypnosis before you get the results you are looking for. Many people will use about 3–4 sessions per area of focus to start seeing significant results. Some people may use up to 8–10 sessions before they experience absolute resolve of the issue that leads them to seek out the power of hypnosis in the first place.

When you are engaged in a hypnosis session, you are essentially relaxing to the point where you can sink deeper into your awareness.

Think of this as being similar to dreaming without actually being asleep.

Through this deep state of relaxation and the ability to sink into your deeper awareness, you can take suggestions from guided meditations and essentially rewire your subconscious mind.

A great example of this is when people use self-hypnosis to encourage themselves to increase their self-esteem. In this case, they introduce positive thoughts about self-esteem and self-confidence to their subconscious minds so that they can begin to have a new mental experience around the topic of themselves.

The Benefits of Hypnotherapy for Weight Loss

It is hard to pinpoint the single best benefit that comes from using hypnosis as a way to engage in weight loss. Hypnosis is a natural, lasting, and deeply impactful weight loss habit that you can use to completely change the way you approach weight loss and food in general for the rest of your life.

With hypnosis, you are not ingesting anything that results in hypnosis working. Instead, you are simply listening to guided hypnosis meditations that help you transform the way your subconscious mind works. As you change your subconscious mind, you will find yourself not even having cravings or unhealthy food urges in the first place.

This means no more fighting against your desires, yo-yo dieting, "falling off the wagon," or experiencing any inner conflict around your eating patterns or your weight loss exercises that are helping you lose the weight.

In addition to hypnosis itself being effective, you can also combine hypnosis with any other weight loss strategy you are using. Changed dietary behaviors, exercise routines, any medications you may be taking with the advisement of your medical practitioner, and any other weight loss practices you may be engaging in can all safely be done with hypnosis. By including hypnosis in your existing weight loss routines, you can improve your effectiveness and rapidly increase the success you experience in your weight loss patterns.

How You Will Lose Weight with Hypnosis

Losing weight with hypnosis works just like any other change with hypnosis will. However, it is important to understand the step by step process so that you know exactly what to expect during your weight loss journey with the support of hypnosis. In general, there are about seven steps that are involved with weight loss using hypnosis. The first step is when you decide to change; the second step involves your sessions; the third and fourth are your changed mindset and behaviors, the fifth step involves your regressions, the sixth is your management routines, and the seventh is your lasting change.

To give you a better idea of what each of these parts of your journey looks like, let's explore them in greater detail below.

In your first step toward achieving weight loss with hypnosis, you have decided that you desire change and that you are willing to try hypnosis as a way to change your approach to weight loss. At this point, you are aware that you want to lose weight, and you have been shown the possibility of losing weight through hypnosis. This is likely the stage you are in right now as you begin reading this very book. You may find yourself feeling curious, open to trying something new, and a little skeptical about whether or not this is going to work for you. You may also be feeling frustrated, overwhelmed, or even defeated by the lack of success you have seen using other weight loss methods, which may be what lead you to seek out hypnosis in the first place. At this stage, the best thing you can do is practice keeping an open and curious mind, as this is how you can set yourself up for success when it comes to your actual hypnosis sessions.

Following your sessions, you are first going to experience a changed mindset. This is where you start to feel far more confident in your ability to lose weight and in your ability to keep the weight off.

At first, your mindset may still be shadowed by doubt, but as you continue to use hypnosis and see your results, you realize that you can create success with hypnosis.

As this evidence starts to show up in your own life, you will find your hypnosis sessions are becoming even more powerful and even more successful.

The final step in your hypnosis journey is going to be the step where you come upon lasting changes. At this point, you are unlikely to need to schedule hypnosis sessions any longer. You should not need to rely on hypnosis at all to change your mindset because you have experienced such significant changes already, and you no longer find yourself regressing into old behaviors. With that being said, you may find that from time to time, you need to have a hypnosis session just to maintain your changes, particularly when an unexpected trigger may arise that may cause you to want to regress your behaviors.

Using Hypnosis to Encourage Healthy Eating and Discourage Unhealthy Eating

As you go through hypnosis to support you with weight loss, there are a few ways that you are going to do so. One of the ways is to focus on weight loss. Another way, however, is to focus on topics surrounding weight loss. For example, you can use hypnosis to encourage yourself to eat healthy while also helping to discourage yourself from unhealthy eating. Effective hypnosis sessions can help you bust cravings for foods that are going to sabotage your success while also helping you feel more drawn to making choices to help you effectively lose weight.

Many people will use hypnosis to change their cravings, improve their metabolism, and even help themselves acquire a taste for eating healthier foods.

You may also use this to encourage you to develop the motivation and energy to prepare healthier foods and eat them so that you are more likely to have these healthier options available.

Using Hypnosis to Encourage Healthy Lifestyle Changes

In addition to helping you encourage yourself to eat healthier while discouraging yourself from eating unhealthy foods, you can also use hypnosis to encourage you to make healthy lifestyle changes. This can support you with everything, from exercising more frequently to picking up more active hobbies that generally support your well-being.

You may also use this to help you eliminate hobbies or experiences from your life that may encourage unhealthy dietary habits in the first place. For example, if you tend to binge eat when you are stressed out, you might use hypnosis to help you navigate stress more effectively so that you are less likely to binge eat when you are feeling stressed out. If you tend to eat when you are feeling emotional or bored, you can use hypnosis to change those behaviors.

Hypnosis can change virtually any area of your life that motivates you to eat unhealthily or otherwise neglect self-care to the point where you are sabotaging yourself from healthy weight loss. It truly is an incredibly versatile practice that you can rely on to help you with weight loss and help you create a healthier lifestyle in general. With hypnosis, there are countless ways that you can improve the quality of your life, making it an incredibly effective practice for you to rely on.

Who Should Try Hypnosis?

Hypnosis is a gentle way for someone to lose weight and create a habit. It isn't a quick fix or a one-time thing. Reframing unhealthy food thinking takes time. Georgia, for example, went eight times a year, and it took a month to begin seeing a real improvement. "The weight fell slowly and gradually, without any drastic adjustments in my lifestyle. I still eat several times a week, but mostly sent food back to me. I enjoyed my food for the first time and had time to drink, taste, and feel the textures. Almost oddly enough, I had to rediscover my love affair with food so that I could lose weight," she says.

The One Downside of Hypnosis for Weight Loss

It is not intrusive; it fits well with other therapies for weight loss and does not require any tablets, powders, or other supplements. Yet there is one downside: quality.

Costs per hour vary but range from $100 to $250 an hour for clinical hypnosis services, and when you see the therapist once or more per week for a month or two, it can add up quickly. And most insurance packages do not support hypnosis. However, it can be compensated if it is included in a broader mental health care program, so consult with your provider.

Best Way to Control Weight Using Hypnosis

Weight management is a lot more than merely slimming down. Healthily managing your weight guarantees ideal health and lowers the risks that come with some diets.

As a result, managing your weight means setting an agreement with yourself to consume healthy and balanced foods in the right quantities, exercising, and minimizing excess body fat.

For these factors, weight management items are becoming equally as popular as weight-loss items.

Guaranteeing you get the appropriate nourishment, correct work-out, and remove dangerous fat from your body can be a lot of work.

With such conflicting recommendations existing in the weight-loss industry, it can be challenging to know when the suggestions you are offered are correct for you, efficient, and in some cases, even safe!

Similarly, when you eat, your body knows when it is complete and sends out signals to your mind informing it so. Many of the time, we disregard these signals and go on consuming!

When you start to listen to your body, it guides you to perform activities, automatically, that keep you in top physical condition!

An individual with a weight problem has often just conditioned their mind to neglect their body!

Through mental training, it is feasible to find out and reverse this scenario to deal with your body so you can achieve your all-natural, suitable weight.

REPLACING THE MIND

The human mind is the most powerful computer system known to man. Your brain and mind are accountable for instantly regulating your heart rate, high blood pressure, and all the other bodily features you take for granted, as well as directing your behaviors, actions, and even your needs. Your mind is a super-computer!

Since your subconscious mind has been conditioned to hate working out, this is what it will do. Because your subconscious mind has been conditioned to believe carrots do not taste good and chocolate tastes fantastic, this is what it will do.

Just as it is feasible to use hypnotherapy to remove anxieties and concerns, it is equally as effortless to use this active mind device to alter your attitude to food and exercise!

DEVELOPING SELF-CONFIDENCE

Over 80% of the world's population is said to suffer from low self-esteem and also an absence of confidence. The world cannot proceed to run well on individuals that have no self-confidence to be leaders and to defend themselves.

I will clarify the significance of self-esteem as well as give useful tips on just how to create confidence, likewise, a positive attitude to ensure that you can start moving toward an extra efficient you.

It is essential to understand what is suggested by "self-esteem" and just how to establish self-confidence. Several people believe that confidence is just conceit or vanity.

Try complying with the confidence pointers noted right here:

CHANGE YOUR THOUGHT PATTERN

Your fight for developing a positive self-image is won in the brain. Adverse thoughts, such as "I can't do this," "I'm most likely going to stop working out again." "I don't have anything useful to fight for" take away your self-confidence and also stop you from even attempting.

To transform your conflicting ideas into favorable ones, firstly, begin by understanding them. Secondly, replace the unfavorable thought. Change the "I'll never be able to do this" to "If I work harder, I think I can do this." When you think about something you cannot do or something you don't like, transform it by thinking about something you can do and declare a positive word.

CREATE A THANKFULNESS LIST

One of the most effective ways to begin changing your self-confidence is to concentrate on the excellent points that you do have in your life, rather than all of the seemingly poor or lacking points. Daily, spend time documenting advantages that occurred to you and things that you have that you are grateful for.

CARE FOR YOURSELF

How we treat our bodies turns into how we consider ourselves. Taking a shower each day, brushing your teeth, combing and making your hair, putting on great clothing that fits you well. Being able to take satisfaction in your appearance will all add to making you feel better as well as more confident concerning your image. Self-care is caring for yourself. You feel better about how you look.

QUIT COMPARING YOURSELF TO OTHERS

With points like social media, we commonly only see the perfect and the greatest successes of our pals. This can make you feel like a failure or like you're not doing things. However, this is not true, as every single person has ups and downs and also struggles. What other individuals are doing or not doing is unimportant? Concentrate on YOUR goals, what matters to YOU.

Spend some time considering it and composing your ideas down if you don't understand what these are. If you attempt to pursue those goals and be satisfied with what you have decided, it matters most.

Training Brain to Burn Fat Fast

Hypnosis has been purported to work very effectively in several different habit-breaking protocols and has undoubtedly been promoted as a good choice for dieters. Is it true? Or is it just another frustrating strategy in a long list of bad approaches to burn the fat faster? Continue reading as I share what I hope is a fresh perspective for you!

If you are open-minded and are ready to believe that the power of the hypnotic idea is real and is going to provide you with a helping hand in your weight loss journey, you are much more likely to see it work.

If you think that hypnosis works and consequently go through hypnosis as a mechanism to assist you to lose weight, you are far more likely to lose weight than a doubter would be.

There are entire bodies of work appearing around this "biology of belief" concept that your inner inclination is the essential element to the success rate you will see when attempting treatments of any kind.

You do need to select an excellent diet plan also! It keeps everybody determined, slimming down, and feeling fantastic.

Bridging the Gap to Success

Hypnosis and weight-loss are a successful pair. Lots of people try to tackle slimming down on their own, merely through self-discipline and motivation, and end up defeated; weight loss hypnosis can supply the missing link that will eventually lead to success. By having the ability to self soothe mentally along with the physical procedure that may be impeding your efforts, hypnotherapists and hypnosis make the entire journey much more accessible, more satisfying, and, eventually, more gratifying.

One needs never to think that it is their fault if they are not able to get down to their preferred weight. Hypnosis and weight loss are a distinct pairing that can tackle our subconscious to assist significantly in losing weight.

When you believe what is involved in the process of losing weight, using hypnosis for weight loss makes a lot of sense. In essence, we are breaking routines, behaviors, beliefs, and desires that we have held firmly for several years. Just thinking of dieting is enough to make anyone feel denied and, therefore, contributes to the level of difficulty that is being experienced.

For that reason, it is essential to discover a way to make the experience simpler and to find out a way to unwind throughout the whole course of dropping weight.

Research study shows that hypnosis, when used correctly, can have a considerable effect when used for weight-loss. A 9-week study of 2 weight management groups—one of which was executing hypnosis as a tool, showed that the group that used hypnosis continued to show results more than two years later on.

Adding hypnosis to any present weight reduction procedures you're currently doing, such as working out and healthy eating, increases your chance of dropping weight by 97%.

Weight-loss is challenging; however, gaining weight is natural. Experts will inform you that a diet plan and exercise is the only way to shed the undesirable pounds; yet, not everyone has the time to sign up with a fitness center, and the stress of life can lead to poor food choices. Hypnosis and weight loss can assist you in developing a more favorable self-image. You will still be you, only better and healthier.

Using hypnosis can help you feel more unwanted and not just about food, but also in your day to day life. When you can conquer stress, you will no longer turn to food for comfort, therefore adopting a much healthier general mindset.

Hypnosis can also help with favorable thinking. You should never underestimate what a positive outlook can attain.

How Successful Is Hypnosis?

The majority of clients require a few sessions of hypnosis for it to have an impact. Many individuals report that they start to reduce weight quickly.

Unfortunately, in the long term, a lot of patients will return to their old habits.

Although they were "taught" how to treat their food, ultimately, they did not decide on their own to deal with food as it should be processed, and they slip back into old methods of overeating.

The answer is that your motivation to modify your habits to decrease or lose excess weight and keep it off must be genuine. No number of Clinical Hypnosis sittings is going to be of any assistance to you if you are not ready yet to do what it takes to lose the weight.

You will discover that, unlike cigarette smoking, we all need food to stay alive, and for almost everybody, eating tasty, fun food is pleasing.

Sadly, what is mouthwatering most of the time is not necessarily excellent for you.

We frequently consume for pleasure, as a kind of satisfaction, centering ourselves on the gustatory feeling as we overgorge with no regard to those signals from our tummy.

However, the truth is, as soon as you eat way too much processed food, you generally don't feel well.

We could use this reality of life as a part of the hypnosis treatment for weight loss. Well, every food is a mix of chemicals that act on our physical structure. We need to recognize that truth to find out how to select foods that work on our body in health-positive and sound methods in order to feel great.

Hypnosis has to do with ideas, and part of it is the posthypnotic idea that deals with you unconsciously when you have an impulse to eat what you acknowledge that you should not to. The particular plans used are customized and developed on the very first examination in the commencement of treatment.

When you had the food, the core of posthypnotic tips is to get you to reroute your attention to how you will feel later on. If the grain produces a lousy feeling once you eat it (and your body currently acknowledges this), your subconscious mind broadcasts to your mindful account a message that effectively specifies: "I do not wish to consume this because I do not wish to feel later on."

This mechanical action to decline things or matters that make us feel bad is imprinted into the subconscious, and with the help of Hypnosis, we learn to deal with or handle such impulses and yearnings. You will also find out brand-new behavioral routines that become automated with the practice of Self-hypnosis.

The usage of posthypnotic tips helps to direct both departments of the mind, conscious and subconscious, for individuals with weight reduction issues, to develop a greater motivation for exercises such as exercise and reduce the number of calories they consume daily to attain their aim for weight reduction.

Furthermore, analytical hypnosis might be used to reveal any prospective unconscious, undesirable emotional sensations that you might be squeezing down with food. In some circumstances, people use food as a means to dull underlying psychological trauma. This needs to be dealt with and resolved.

THE USE OF FOOD IS NOT MEANT TO BE AN ANESTHETIC

A couple of sessions of hypnosis with a qualified therapist can cause favorable cognitive procedures. To discover self-hypnosis the proper way, the most efficient thing to do is to have some Person-to-person hypnosis sittings with a qualified, scientific hypnosis professional in his/her office. By using self-hypnosis, you can help yourself so that you can preserve your weight loss objectives, correct weight, and recover your health.

ATTEMPT IT AT HOME

If you can't manage hypnotherapy or simply aren't comfy working with a hypnotherapist, you can carry out hypnotherapy on your own.

After a week or more, the statements you've been listening to will begin to change the chatter in your head and ideally assist you in making healthier decisions with less of a conscious battle.

How Hypnosis Clears the Metabolic Programming That Prevents Weight Loss

If you are overweight, you may be sick of reminding people that losing weight means consuming less food and getting fewer calories. You may have tried both old and new diets. Yet it also seems that our bodies have found a way to turn a lettuce plate into a pound of fat! Many people who want to lose weight sooner or later find out that aerobic systems keep their weight on the body regardless of whether their eating patterns change and hinder their efforts.

If you or your friend or client is overweight, and you want to see how these services impact weight loss efforts, take the following questionnaire:

- Should you eat less than your slim mates to lose weight?
- Are you thinking of food cravings just when the pounds start to fall off? As if you were hungry rather than dietary?
- Are you exhausted and lethargic while you diet?
- Do you find that the weight doesn't fall as fast as it should, no matter how much you starve?
- Are you gaining all your weight back from an alarming-speed diet?
- If you replied "yes" to one of these questions, you probably have a subconscious metabolism that retains your body weight instead of consuming it for energy.

Here are the good ones now! There are several ways we can approach this system by hypnosis to start battling the body and food cravings to lose weight!

First, the possible causes of this programming must be investigated.

The metabolism of food is the dynamic mechanism by which the body absorbs and uses nutrients from food. This is a dynamic mechanism involving a variety of variables. One is the thyroid gland feature, the 'master' switch that controls the cell metabolism levels.

Via hypnotic imaging, the main metabolic hormone released by the thyroid gland, thyroxine, is released. More thyroxine means more fat has been consumed, and more energy has been lost to you. There may be medical causes for thyroid dysfunction, but before going into hypnotherapy, we recommend a full physical evaluation and a potential check for thyroid function.

The development of two main pancreatic hormones, insulin and glucagons, is another essential factor in body metabolism processes. Such primary metabolic hormones hold or burn our body fat. The foods you consume affect the activities of these hormones directly. In general, most carbohydrates, including sugars, tend to cause insulin secretion, which increases the metabolism of sugar and storage. Glucagons, which are secreted after a low-carbon meal, allow the body to consume protein and fat, including fat stores of the body. This is part of why low carb diets are popular.

So How Does Hypnosis Help You Change Your Eating Choices?

Since all eating habits are ingrained in the unconscious, consciously choosing to eat differently is rarely enough to make changes in our food habits in the long term. The image of hypnosis targets and adjusts these subconscious programs in a way that is both stable and almost straightforward.

Personal hypnotic scripts that can be written on a self-hypnosis tape and heard in bed every night can be produced by working with a hypnotherapist.

Exercise is also an essential component of metabolism activation.

Studies have discovered that daily exercise not only speeds up metabolism during the workout but even for hours after, even when you rest, even if you exercise as little as 30 minutes a day. Of course, many of us have trouble exercising. Join the power of hypnosis again. Hypnotic ideas can be used to improve motivation and strength, and stamina for physical activity. Most times, it takes even more to get interested in exercise than simple hypnotic advice.

Some of the creative methods we use will lead you back to what you liked to do as a child. You can choose one or two of the activities you will enjoy again! We use the power of hypnosis to bring back your excitement as a child. We can also go back to these painful encounters, which have made us turn to the joys of physical activity to save the past from these traumas. For example, an experience of being rejected, humiliated, or hurt on the playground in a team sport may cause one to avoid playing outside. Our rescue mission enables the child to receive comfort and promise of self-assurance from an adult and an invitation to play with the adult on the outside.

Genetics is one of the most common sources of metabolic programming. Some human genetics (South Pacific Islanders and Eskimos are only two extreme examples) retain fat more readily on their bodies because, for thousands of years in particular during famines, these traits have served their forefathers well. It is impossible for even qualified clinicians to alter certain genetic codes in our DNA. We may, however, convince the metabolism to bypass these DNA programs through hypnosis and help us lose fat. Once my clients told me, "My whole family is overweight." Now is the time to use such hypnotic techniques to bypass DNA programming.

Another common concern with those dealing with weight loss is that the subconscious mind can fear weight loss, and if weighing concerns are absent, even scarier issues will potentially be experienced.

7

The Change

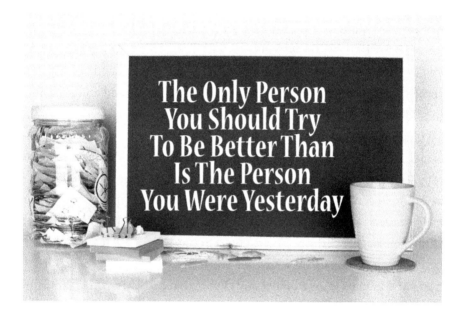

Creating the Right Mindset

CHOOSE A MANTRA OR SET OF MANTRAS THAT MOTIVATE YOU

You can create a slogan or use a quote yourself. Create a habit of saying your mantra aloud during the day at scheduled times, like getting up, lunch, or just before bedtime. Posting the mantras is also helpful.

Good mantras include "every day is a new beginning and an opportunity for progress," "I am strong, powerful and able to accomplish my objectives," and "I can accomplish them if I think so."

You can use simple notes like post-it notes to display your mantras, or you can use art prints. Put them in your refrigerator, in your mirror toilet, or on your house walls. Pick a place you can see them every day.

USE POSITIVE SELF-TALK

Everybody has an internal voice, not always friendly. But turning that voice into a positive can improve your life. You can do this by catching and reframing negative thoughts positively. Besides, tell yourself about you, your future, and your goals consciously.

Your mind can say to you, for example, "You're not well enough." You may turn around and say, "I'm good enough, but sometimes I get frustrated with the challenges. Things will look different tomorrow."

In general, say things to yourself like, "I am proud of myself for working hard every day," "I've done a lot, and the best things are yet to come," and, "I know that I can do this if I continue to work hard."

REFRAME ACTIVITIES THAT YOU DON'T ENJOY

It is normal not to enjoy your journey to your destination. You may love your work, but you hate parts of your workday, or you may want to have a cross country marathon but hate hills. You can shift your vision by imagining it dimming and then incorporating new emotions. Imagine, for example, your stress on deadlines is gone, then imagine how good you feel when you complete a project.

Focus on the aspects you enjoy or benefit from these activities. For starters, it may be hard to walk hills, but it also provides you with a better view of the countryside.

One way to do this is to concentrate on what you do and feel while you do not enjoy the activities.

You may hate working meetings, for example, but concentrate on changing the landscape, talking with your fellow workers, or making a good impression on your boss.

CONNECT WITH OTHERS WHO SHARE YOUR GOALS

Make friends on a journey like you or join a group for like-minded people. They can be terrific motivators to keep track of it and can even be useful in times of difficulty.

Look for like-minded friends in your destination online or in places. For example, to meet other aspiring musicians, you could attend an open mic night.

You can also search for groups on websites like meetup.com.

Don't waste time with those who take you down. Choose the motivators instead.

COMPARE YOURSELF TO PAST YOU, NOT OTHERS

It is so tentative to compare yourself with others, but it is always an error. Regardless of how well you do, you always rank second. It is better to connect yourself to you! Remember where you have been in the past and now. Try to be better than you were before.

When you catch yourself comparing yourself to others, remember that you will most probably see their highlights—not every day's nitty-gritty details.

Make a list of your positive features and achievements to remember how far you have already gone!

MAKE A GRATITUDE LIST

By recognizing everything you must thank, you can create the positive attitude you need to remain motivated. Write down all the good things in your life, especially the things you have worked hard to get. Post your list somewhere you can see it, for example, on the fridge or lock screen of your telephone.

It is best to make lists of gratitude often. You could even write down three to five items for which you are grateful every day.

Over time, the appreciation list will make you feel better about life, helping to increase your drive to continue focusing on what is important to you.

Working Towards Goals

KEEP YOUR GOALS SMALL AND MEASURABLE

It's cool to have big ambitions but to make them easier to achieve; you have to work on them. Break the bigger objectives into smaller ones. Then identify parameters for evaluating them.

Similarly, the major goal might be to run a marathon. You could set a small goal to run a 5K. You can calculate this aim by measuring how far you go every day or by registering for a race.

CREATE AN ACTION PLAN FOR YOUR GOALS

You can build an ambitious strategy to meet your big objective, or you can limit it to your specific objectives. Include what you want to do, what you are going to do, and how you evaluate your success.

For example, your big goal might be to run the marathon, and your small objectives could be to run a mile, 5K, 10K, and run a half marathon.

Don't get stuck in the details. Write out a basic framework for your action plan and then work towards your objectives. You can modify or add to the scheme later.

Keep it brief with a short description. You don't have to prepare all the details. For example, you can start your marathon action plan by focusing on the steps you must take to run a full mile, including purchasing new shoes, downloading a running app, and running three times a week.

DISPLAY YOUR ACTION PLAN WHERE YOU CAN SEE IT EVERY DAY

You can post it at home, place it in your calendar, or make it your digital wallpaper. See if you're on target every day. Often, it's all right to get behind; however, your action plan will keep you on track.

Try to place your strategy on the fridge.

Also, at work, if you are allowed to.

Choose a position that you can conveniently look at.

TRACK YOUR PROGRESS

Seeing how far you have come can be a great motivator! Keep track of all the milestones, whether large or small. Just one step towards your target is a success, so give credit to yourself!

- Write down all your achievements so that when you feel discouraged, you can read about them.
- You can even visually remember your development.
- You could put up a poster with a trail on it if your target is to run a marathon.

Divide the trail into 26.2 different parts. Whenever you increase your target, color in a different segment.

REWARD YOURSELF FOR HARD WORK AND PERSISTENCE

Rewards motivate you to keep up with your goal. Choose an enticing reward for you. Consider something that helps you to accomplish your goals, if possible. Here are some fantastic thoughts:

You could be rewarded by sticking to the goal of writing every day, with a new notebook.

Get a massage that will reward you for meeting your goals.

You can enjoy a special meal with friends that helped you achieve your goal.

Treat yourself to a bubble bath.

You can celebrate your kickboxing success (or other sport) by buying a pair of new weight gloves.

A relaxing yoga session.

Time to read a good book.

DO SOMETHING YOU ENJOY EVERY DAY

Just working towards something that you enjoy can be daunting, so take your time. Please spend at least a few minutes per day enjoying yourself, whether it is an episode of a favorite television show or a favorite treat, or coffee with a friend. This helps you to stay motivated when times get rough.

PREPARE YOURSELF FOR SETBACKS

Setbacks are part of life, and all of them happen. They're not saying you're a loser! Create a quick outline of how you can conquer any challenges and know that you can.

For instance, you may want to talk to a friend, take a day to brainstorm solutions, and then complete a small task to help you achieve your goal.

Inform yourself, "Everything is part of the trip. As I have conquered them in the past, I will conquer this challenge."

Beating Procrastination

SPEND TIME WORKING ON YOUR GOAL EVERY DAY

If you are working successfully towards your goal, the body releases dopamine, the hormone that makes you take action. Fortunately, with even a small amount of progress, you can increase your dopamine. Even if you can work only for 15 minutes on a certain day to reach your goal, you can see results.

AVOID OVERTHINKING ABOUT YOUR WORK AND GOALS

Too much thought can be detrimental for two reasons. First, it keeps you in your head and prevents you from acting. Furthermore, it allows you to worry about future issues that will possibly never happen. When you get lost in your thoughts, take action, begin with a small mission. You will be back on track when you check the mission.

When you begin to overthink, write down your thoughts, then try to draw up a to-do list so you can concentrate.

You may not be able to deal with all your problems today, but some progress can be made.

BUILD YOUR ROUTINES AROUND YOUR GOALS

If you work on personal or professional goals, routines are important. Get used to setting aside time blocks to complete the activities you need to do.

For example, get up every day early to focus on your task, like going for an early morning run or working on your novel for an hour.

Every day start your workday the same way. For example, you could review your to-do list for the easiest things that day, answer e-mail messages, or develop a regular action plan.

Develop a routine after lunch that helps you get on track again. For example, after lunch, you might arrange all your meetings to help you get back on track immediately.

TAKE CONTROL OVER YOUR SCHEDULE

People and other activities can take part of your time. It's up to you to adjust your life and make sure you have time for it all. It means that you often have to say "no" to certain things to make room for others. Don't live your life as others like—spend your time doing what is important to you.

Plan meetings for you to achieve personal goals. You can also do things that make you content with this time.

LEARN TO SAY "NO" TO THINGS YOU DON'T WANT TO DO

It's all right to say no without guilt when someone asks for your time and conflicts with working towards your goal. Set your time limits and practice saying "no" to strangers. When the time comes, praise the individual and then turn it down gently.

Say, "Your Halloween party sounds like a lot of fun, but that day I have already committed to something."

You don't need to explain why, so don't feel pressured to justify your decision.

ASK FOR HELP IF YOU NEED IT

Sometimes you may be discouraged because you have had problems such as a hard task or lack of resources. Ask for help when this happens! Often someone can support you.

For example, you could ask your flatmate to stop slacking off and clean the house.

You could ask your running buddies to come with you and train.

You could borrow a piece of equipment you need from a friend that has it.

Overcoming Psychological Blocks to Weight Loss

There could be a psychological block in your way if you've tried every diet and exercise plan and can't slim down. Weight loss is an up-hill battle for all, but emotional fights will take a longer time to reach their goals. The first step towards a safe solution is to recognize the problem. You may find there is more than one roadblock. The good news, however, is that these challenges can be resolved.

THE LINK BETWEEN EMOTIONS AND WEIGHT LOSS

Most of us have good intentions to eat better and exercise more often. And most of us know the essential things are to eat and to stop. Yet we still end up derailing our progress when we feel tired, anxious, bored, or irritated even with our best intentions. And let's face it, these feelings often keep popping up.

We are creatures of habit. Comfort is contained within our routine. And, naturally, you search for such comfortable routines when your routine involves diet and activity patterns that have contributed to weight gain. Such patterns relieve discomfort—at least in the short term.

What's worse, you probably have strong rational skills to sustain unhealthy habits. After all, why should you consider practicing relaxation and comfort?

It is especially difficult to change our behaviors in the case of food behaviors. Our bodies are meant for eating. And when we do, we feel better. But not everything is lost if you want to change your weight loss habits. Weight loss counseling works somehow against you, but it can work for you as it has for others. Before getting around the roadblock, you may need to find out what the roadblock is.

COMMON PSYCHOLOGICAL BLOCKS TO WEIGHT LOSS AND MAINTENANCE

These are the most common emotional problems when people struggle to slim down. Check the list to see if something looks familiar.

All-or-Nothing Thinking

If you walk a fine line between completely sticking to your food plan or falling off the road, you might encounter a cognitive distortion called all or nothing. The term "cognitive distortion" is used by psychologists to mean persistently exaggerated thoughts that do not conform to what happens in the real world.

People who experience all or nothing when trying to lose weight think that their food choices are either a complete success or a total failure. Research has shown that a thought-style of something or nothing is closely related to a perceived lack of control over food and an inability to maintain a healthy weight. Some researchers have compared this lack of control to the actions of Jekyll and Hyde.

Unless you do not think so, you usually struggle with a little indulgence to return to a balanced eating schedule. Then, you would simply throw your towel and overeat because your diet has failed anyway.

Negative Body Image

If you try to change the size of your body and its shape, you may be less than satisfied with the current way it looks. Of course, there's nothing wrong with improving your health or appearance. But if your body image is too negative, the weight loss process can be impeded.

Researchers have demonstrated that in those who are obese, body dissatisfaction is more common than in those who are normal in weight. A negative corporal image is also associated with unhealthy eating patterns and other problems. For example, weight and shape concerns can also be embarrassing and lead to avoidance of self-consciousness and excessive feelings of fatness after eating.

It is not clear whether a bad body image leads to unhealthy food or whether unhealthy food leads to a negative body image. What is clear is that a strong dissatisfaction with your body can prevent you from maintaining a healthy weight.

Stress

There's a good reason for the name of comfort food. Most people feel good about eating. And some people use food as the best way to calm their emotions during times of stress.

Although it is common in people of all sizes and forms, this strategy can create problems if you are trying to lose weight.

Studies have found that excessive consumption can become a chronic management mechanism for stressful lives. The strategy may be more common among the overweight.

And it's not just excessive food that can be problematic. Your food choices will probably change if you feel more anxious. Research published in Physiology and Behavior found that we eat more not only when depressed, but also we target foods that are usually avoided when we are trying to lose weight or for health reasons.

Depression

Studies are not sure whether depression induces weight gain or whether depression prevents loss of weight. Yet many scientists think there's a link. And even among people with average weight, depression can be troublesome in weight terms. Evidence has indicated that over-weight perception raises psychological distress and can contribute to depression.

Symptoms associated with depression, such as sleeplessness or inac-tivity, may make weight loss harder. And some widely prescribed anti-depressants can also contribute to weight gain.

Personal or Childhood Trauma

Several studies have found that people at higher risk of obesity are vulnerable to physical violence, sexual harassment, or peer bullying. Those with emotional trauma can change their eating habits to the de-gree that they affect their weight. Some scientists suggest that weight gain can be used for survivors of violence as an emotionally safe "solu-tion."

Not everyone with personal or childhood traumas struggles to keep their weight stable. Yet there may be a link if you have witnessed vio-lence, neglect, or bullying.

Tips to Overcome Barriers

You might have found that you are familiar with one or more of the common psychological barriers to weight loss. It is not unusual to face multiple barriers on a healthy journey. However, these roadblocks do not have to prevent your success.

Each of the following tips and suggestions will overcome many ob-stacles. These suggestions are also healthy wellness strategies that have no side effects and are almost entirely free. Consider trying to find one or more of these solutions.

KEEP A JOURNAL

Stress avoidance is not always possible. However, you can identify and do your best to avoid certain situations or people that undermine your success. Maintaining a food journal can be helpful. Also, research has shown that maintaining a food journal can double the effects of weight loss.

Are you overeating or eating unhealthy food in certain environments or around certain people? Can you identify certain situations that make you feel out of control and uncomfortable? A journal will help you assess these circumstances so you can restrict or fully prevent your exposure.

MAKE SMALL CHANGES

When you think something is all or nothing that keeps you from adhering to your food schedule. Consider taking small steps and setting short-term goals.

Second, find a positive transition that is fair and achievable. You can walk every day for 15 minutes after dinner. Sets a goal for a week to focus on this goal. If you keep a food log, write down each day's information on various ways you have achieved in moving the goal forward.

Note, success is not your goal, but any effort to step in the right direction is progress, of which you must be proud.

LISTEN TO SELF-TALK

Watch out for the messages you send to yourself all day long? These recurrent thoughts can create a roadblock to good weight loss.

Many that are susceptible to a negative view of their body will find themselves hearing negative messages about their body every day. Phrases such as "I'm so fat" or "I'm so out of shape" spoken loudly or loudly in your head that weaken your ability to make a healthier move when the opportunity is there.

Listen to your inner conversation for a week or two. Identify a message or two that can encourage a negative self-image. Replace these messages with a mighty mantra. Phrases such as "My body is strong," "I'm strong enough," or "I have come a long way" are widely used to build confidence.

LEARN RELAXATION TECHNIQUES

If you cannot avoid difficult individuals or environments, relaxation strategies can be a safe alternative to emotional control in stressful situations.

Researchers have found that a particular kind of relaxation technique, known as guided imaging, can help with weight loss. You should work with a therapist to learn directed imagery, but guided imagery can also be learned by yourself.

This takes time for you to learn, but controlled imaging can be the most powerful tool for weight loss in stressful times if your emotions cause you to overeat.

PRIORITIZE SLEEP

Studies have consistently found that sleep patterns are related to stress, depression, and poor eating behaviors. So, changing your bedtime routine is one of the simplest, most effective moves to overcome psychological obstacles.

Consider your bedroom a sleeping sanctuary. Disable electronics (TV, monitor, cell phone) and do whatever you can to minimize noise. Get light-blocking sheets or buy a sleep mask so that the night is completely dark. Many people also raise the thermostat to facilitate restful sleep. Try to go to bed every night and wake up every morning at the same time.

SEEK HELP

Most professionals are specially qualified to deal with stress, past trauma, and other issues that may impede successful weight loss. A mental health professional can address the underlying emotional causes of alcohol, overeating, and weight gain.

Your doctor may be in a position to provide a referral. There are other ways to find a therapist, if not.

The American Psychological Association offers resources to help consumers find practitioners in your area, including a local guide.

If you do not see a behavioral health professional in your area, you can use an online platform such as email, Skype, or facetime for your mental health consultation. These therapy services often provide much-needed relief.

STAY MOTIVATED FOR WEIGHT LOSS

Staying motivated is crucial to complete your weight loss program successfully. Often, in the first week of your weight loss program, you are very excited and do whatever you can to lose weight. You go to the gym; you change your eating habits, and you get up early in the morning and go for a walk. The first week goes great.

In the second week, your old habits win over your new habits. You go to a lunchroom with your colleagues and can't prevent yourself from eating those juicy burgers and pizzas. You won't even feel like going to the gym. You show idleness in getting up early in the morning as well.

Why does all this happen? We are super excited in the first few weeks, and then in the next few weeks, all our energy and excitement vanish, and we finally give up.

The answer is simple. It's all because of a lack of motivation. We are super motivated in the first week of our weight loss endeavor. Inspiration prompts vitality and fervor, which encourages us to do all that we can to lose weight. In any case, in the subsequent week, our inspiration begins to back off, and, accordingly, we want to stop, surrender, and return to our old habits.

It's all because of low motivation that most people often quit on their weight loss program. You can keep yourself motivated during rough spots using motivational quotes.

Tips and Advice to Motivate Yourself to Lose Weight

When you want to lose weight, one of the main difficulties is to find the motivation to do so. How many of us have embarked on regimes that we did not keep for lack of real motivation or sufficient strength of character to face this challenge? Losing weight is not trivial, and above all, it is not easy. More often than not, having a lack of motivation has more to do with the structure of our weight loss program than with the mentality that we have.

ASK YOURSELF THE RIGHT QUESTIONS

Before embarking on a weight loss program, you will have to ask yourself why you are doing it—a simple question, which many do not ask.

It usually happens that we start a diet after a comment a loved one made. Maybe your mother tells you that you should be a bit careful about what you eat. You may also be triggered after looking at a magazine with skinny, stunning women and wanting to look like that.

But if you want to lose weight effectively, you have to do it for yourself. And to keep your motivation to lose weight, you have to be highly interested! If you realize that you are not doing it for yourself, it will undoubtedly be more difficult to stick to your diet because of someone else.

On the other hand, if you decide to regain control and eliminate your extra pounds for good reasons (aesthetics, health, and more), and all these are important to you, then you are already on a good path.

THINK ABOUT THE NEGATIVE CONSEQUENCES

When you have low motivation and want to snack or eat something unhealthy, you are too lazy to do your workout.

Rather than thinking about the positive sides of the action: instant satisfaction, eating something sweet, staying quiet at home, etc., think of the negative consequences: we are going to screw up a day of effort, we will take more time to reach our objectives, we will have to make efforts for longer, etc.

IMAGINE REALIZING YOUR NEW HABITS

No matter what project you want to do, it's all about habits. And in the end, it is they who make all the difference.

The problem with habits is that we have to manage to incorporate them sustainably into our daily lives. To do this, you have to imagine yourself carrying out the actions that make up this habit. The more details, the more effective it will be.

When you have the idea of a habit that will help you advance your project, imagine yourself carrying it out. So, when the real-time comes to perform this action, you will have no more problems since your brain will already be prepared to perform it; it will already be somewhat used to it.

COMPARE THE TWO POSSIBLE FUTURES

To achieve what you want to achieve, you have to make the right choices. Easy to say, but day after day, it is hard not to crack. And that's why we have to project ourselves into the future.

When one is faced with a desire or the contrary, it is necessary to compare the two possible futures. See yourself in the future situation when you make the wrong choice and the one where you make the right choice.

Imagine the consequences of your actions, and you will see that you will always make the right decision. This little exercise will help you take action when necessary and not crack when you are subjected to temptation.

UNDERSTAND THAT IT IS ONLY STARTING THAT IS DIFFICULT

It is always the beginning, the start, which is the most difficult.

Who hasn't said to himself at the gym: "Damn, it pisses me off to be here!"

Who hasn't said to himself after cooking a healthy dish: "It annoys me to eat that."

On the contrary, we are happy and proud to have moved and to have accomplished something during our day. In reality, all the difficulty is in starting. Once we have passed that, it's easy; everything is done on its own, without effort.

So, keep that in mind when you are becoming a little lazy: you have already done the most difficult part. If you pass this test, the rest will flow calmly.

ALWAYS KEEP YOUR GOALS IN MIND

Regardless of what you do, there is at least one reason why you do it: your goals.

And these goals are doubly important. First, they help you define the actions you will need to take to get there. Second, they will help you stay motivated for the time it takes to complete your projects.

And that's why you have to keep them in mind, visualize them well. Because when you have lower motivation, you can remember these goals. And they will help you to hold on, to cope. And then, you will be much more likely to make the right choice.

ORGANIZE TO OVERCOME PROCRASTINATION

Procrastination is everyone's enemy. It is what blocks us in almost everything we want to achieve in life. Fortunately for us, there are ways to short-circuit it.

The first thing to understand is that it is normal to tend to procrastinate. It comes from the very structure of our brain—so no need to feel sad.

The second thing to understand is that if procrastination is more and more present, it is because it is linked to concentration.

And as we are constantly called upon by our smartphones, our notifications, our emails, etc., we find it harder and harder to concentrate.

START LIGHT

What makes a project successful in the long run? It is often a balance between attendance and intensity, but people tend to favor intensity over attendance.

Wrongly!

What will make a difference, in the long run, is attendance.

The intensity of your hypnosis does not matter.

If you do not keep at it continuously and effectively, you will not have lasting results.

On the contrary, if you make small changes, and you keep these changes precise over time, you will have significant results.

That's why you have to start light.

Think regularity and long term rather than intensity.

Start with new habits and gradually incorporate others.

CELEBRATE

From time to time, you have to know how to release the pressure and start on the right foot.

You have to know how to realize that you are accomplishing something great and that what you are doing is something few people manage.

And so, you have to know how to celebrate your efforts. Enjoy yourself and be proud of what you accomplish daily. Be careful not to abuse it; it could be counterproductive.

DON'T WAIT TO BE MOTIVATED TO TAKE ACTION

This is a mistake made by most people. They are convinced that they must be motivated to take action. When, in reality, motivation comes from the action itself. To motivate yourself, act.

You will see that the more you do, however small, the more you will feel proud and confident in your ability to achieve. And the more you will be motivated to make new ones.

Focus on what you gain, not what you lose.

The purpose of this tip is to appreciate the changes rather than lament their difficulty.

To do this, you have to think positively. Please focus on the positive aspects that this change will bring you rather than the negative aspects that result from this change.

And all the more so when you know that it is the start that is the most difficult. Because positive thinking will allow you to make this start easier, and behind it, it goes on quietly.

DON'T BE ALONE

When you are alone, it is not easy to get active every day and do things every day.

When you embark on a project, I strongly advise you to embark with another person. Moving with others will allow you to cope with reduced motivation easily because you will not have these drops in motivation at the same time as others. When it is necessary to move, it will be easier as others will push you to do it. Thus, we motivate each other—a truly virtuous circle.

LIFESTYLE SHIFT

The motivation to lose weight can easily be sustained as a result of allowing yourself to live in an "unconstrained" manner of existence. A lifestyle change is not the same as dieting. Thus, it gives a more relaxed transitional period than throwing yourself into programs centered around dreaded calorie counting and scales.

Instead, dropping weight can become a more fulfilling process than simply reaching an ultimate target weight. By allowing your mind to be in sync with your body, you can naturally (but not without dedicated effort) alter your perception of food, exercise, and dieting. Remember, however, that change is not easy, but it also does not have to be a tug-of-war between where you want to go and where you are present.

MAKE A PLEDGE TO GET HEALTHY

By striving toward a positive and fit lifestyle, you can enjoy the things you like but just in moderation. Depriving yourself of the food items you love will only lead to self-defeat because restrictions rarely allow a person to flourish.

As soon as you have decided to lose weight and pursue a healthy lifestyle, it would help if you make a promise to yourself to remain true to good health. It can also be useful to enlist friends or close relatives to help keep you focused on your targets when times get a little tougher. You can both embark on this voyage of health with each other as partners and take control of your weight. Either way, becoming healthier is what is most important.

MOTIVATE YOURSELF WITH THE RESULTS!

What better motivation to lose weight can we find than that offered by the mirror or others' gaze?

The more effective your diet, the more you will want to continue. You will be delighted to see the weight drop on the scale, see that others look at you differently or compliment you, and see your figure change in the mirror. It is good that you give yourself so much trouble!

What if things don't go as fast as expected? No worries, favor the positive! Even if you've lost less weight than expected, it's still lost. And if you find that your figure is not yet as you would like, tell yourself that you are on the right track.

It is important to tell you that it is a quest, sometimes a long-term one, which will pay off at one time or another. If your weight is not yet impacted, know that you are doing your body and your body good in any case!

REWARD YOUR SMALL ACHIEVEMENTS

Another way of finding the motivation to lose weight during the trials and tribulations is to take the time to reward yourself for the little goals you have accomplished. As opposed to withholding from celebrating until you have achieved the goal of losing 100 lbs. (which is anything but a small feat), instead reward yourself for easier, more short-term goals while going along the way toward your ultimate destination. Doing so will ensure you keep thinking positive and on the path to success.

BE ACTIVE

Staying active is the primary factor in weight loss. Giving yourself difficult but realistic health exercises like taking the stairs or walking to work, challenging yourself within reason is an excellent way to increase stamina and self-esteem. The more you put yourself to the test, the more complex your fitness targets become, and the more exercise and activity will become a habit for you within your daily routine.

How to Heal Your Body

What does your body tell you in your own life of the need to heal the wound? Every day, the body sends out signals which let you know how safe it really is in general. Aches and pains are usually a warning somewhere deep inside that something is wrong. Some of the origins are a little more obvious than others. It is up to you to take the time to listen to the hints about your overall health that your body offers.

POSITIVE THOUGHT

Nearly every religion in the world states that positive thinking plays a significant role in healing.

When it is a necessity for you to heal the body, it is a good idea to spend a little time thinking each day positively.

You may just find that in this age-old philosophy, you have made a believer out of yourself in no time when you start to experience the power of positive thinking working inside your body to build a healthier you.

EXERCISE

Exercise is one of the most neglected factors in healing the body. Over the years, it has been reduced to a fitness role and is equated with the need to keep in shape or assist in that goal rather than a balanced practice in and of itself. Exercise releases endorphins to provide relief from pain and a sense of happiness and well-being at large.

GOOD DIET

A balanced diet is a wonderful resource for healing your body as much as it can pain you to know it. To maintain maximum health, you need other nutrients.

Unfortunately, we live in a world of fast food, and very few people get the nutrients required for optimum health. That's why it's important to bear in mind other choices like vitamin supplements—although they're not nearly as successful as getting the nutrients through your diet.

ADOPT HEALTHY HABITS

There are some behaviors that you can adopt that will promote improved health.

Replace antibacterial soap with your regular hand soap. Wash your hands often and wash them well. Teach your family how to wash their faces, cover their mouths, and use sanitizing hand wipes or liquid cleaners in public to reduce the risk of taking home infections and diseases. Such practices can seem too simplistic but will keep you safe and protected, allowing the body to heal.

PROTECTING THE BODY WITH HYPNOSIS

Self-hypnosis is just another means of protecting the body from illnesses of all kinds. Many ways mastering the art of self-hypnosis can help in your struggle, whether you are trying to handle a cancer diagnosis or ward off the common cold.

Hypnosis can help you relax, open your mind to positive thinking, help the nutrients get where they are best served, and help boost immunity, among other great things.

TAKE CONTROL OF YOUR HEALING PROCESS

It is time for you to take control of your body and its process of healing. Whether you are using one or all of the above techniques, if you listen to your body and react accordingly—for the best possible health outcome—you can find real help when it comes to healing the body.

Hypnosis is a powerful mode that literally can help your body stop unwanted habits and then start to heal and rejuvenate your body. It's all about the computer device situated within the brain.

Stress creates the need to smoke, or does it cause stress? It is very difficult to go cold-turkey in this modern-day world where tension is a daily occurrence. Hypnotherapy is often the last option, and yet hypnotherapy for smoking cessation is the most successful strategy. More so than any prescription medication designed to quit smoking.

Stress will manifest itself in all sorts of scenarios, ranging from being depressed to violent.

Contrary to common opinion, medications just exacerbate the condition while making huge bucks for the pharmaceuticals. Seek your nearest hypnotherapist first before you go to get medication to be healthy again. You're going to be happier faster, and it's going to last a lot longer!

Will they hypnotize you? The condition you strive to achieve is one of absolute relaxation as though you're about to fall asleep. You are still very much in charge because we are enhancing your drive to do what you set out to do.

Hypnosis is essentially a form of deep relaxation that allows the client to take an imagined journey. The imagination is where you build a new, vibrant vision for what you want to be like in your future.

When your critical mind is in a very deep relaxed state, it calms down from that constant thinking that says: "I can't just leave," or "It's just too hard to quit." Side-stepping the critical mind lets you become motivated to accomplish what you felt was impossible before. Not only does it work well with smoking, but it also works well in sports, handling discomfort, and even taking exams.

Old habits of thinking can be replaced quickly and lovingly with fresh, wonderful optimistic thoughts that can leave such a positive force in your life.

Imagine if you can avoid obsessing about a question, you can actually do anything, or be, or have anything. You broke the habit, and you can achieve anything you set out to do. Your level of confidence can reach the sky!

The most common problem is that after quitting smoking, customers assume they'll gain weight. When the body recovers from the smoking effects, it could lead to a weight loss or gain. It is a positive thing showing that the body is in the healing process. You can also eradicate the habit with hypnosis and stop replacing one oral obsession with another.

The subconscious mind is already planting the new thought cycle, and when you listen to your private session's mp3, you can really reduce the weight tension.

I suggest that you choose a hypnotherapist who guides you to rejuvenate your heart and lungs back to an age you feel tremendous strength and energy. A successful hypnotherapist can even get your liver to detoxify your body very gently so that the tar and nicotine or even heavy metals can be extracted very quickly and easily. The body is in the healing process and will remain there for a few months.

Hypnotherapy will help move the body into new wellness. Your cells can be ordered to heal through the science of epigenetics.

Hypnosis is the best way to help cancer patients help the body cure at faster speeds, particularly with surgeries. Studies that show hypnosis heals the body have been performed to minimize bleeding, swelling, and bruises, as well as speed up the recovery process to 10 times faster. In addition to that, it has been established that 10 minutes of hypnosis actually reduces blood pressure and lowers cholesterol.

If you want to quit smoking, eradicate a phobia, help heal cancer or pain, then just use your strong and focused mind to seek it out without medication. It is a lot easier than you could ever imagine. You become a champion, and you'll be shocked by how strong you are.

Stay Conscious, Maintain Your Changes
DIETS END, HEALTH DOESN'T

Experts have long said that to keep weight off, people need to make long-term changes to their diet and activity levels. Remember that slow but steady wins the race. According to the CDC, those who lose weight at a pace of one to two pounds per week tend to keep weight off more successfully. Further, they emphasize how important it is to take steps to ensure you maintain your weight loss.

Hypnosis is different from normal "diets" because it doesn't promote temporary change. Hypnotherapy helps you resist going back to your old ways, but that doesn't mean that you don't also need to keep up your efforts. Hypnosis instills a tendency towards long term change, but if you don't fight to keep that change up, you're going to go back to how you were. Accordingly, take the messages you learn through hypnosis and reinforce them as much as you can after you've finished hypnotherapy. You can continue to use scripts on your own if you want to ensure that you maintain progress.

Too many people return to their original weights after they lose weight. Only about ten to twenty percent of people keep weight off and don't return to their original weight or higher after losing weight.

This weight is often regained within five years, or sometimes in as little time as just weeks, depending on how much you've lost. Thus, if you don't remain conscious of your habits, you may start to incorporate the ones that you'd ditched.

Carry all the changes you've made through even after you've stopped hypnotherapy.

You probably won't want to continue hypnotherapy forever, but you need to keep up with all the dietary, physical, and mental changes that you've made on this journey because they are vital to your overall well-being and happiness. Don't let this journey end by returning to who you were. Continue on your path of growth.

You have to continue fighting for your health, and when you're stressed or anxious, doing this may get hard, but there's no end to maintaining your health. That is something that you'll have to do for the rest of your life. You cannot avoid the effort required to maintain your new weight, but it does get easier over time. You get used to the changes, and the changes eventually feel so natural that they are incredibly easy to keep up with.

DON'T FORGET WHAT YOU'VE FOUGHT FOR

Never forget the effort you put in once you got to your goal weight.

You need to remember the time and energy you invested so that you feel motivated not to go back. You don't want to have to start all over and do that work again after you worked so hard to make progress. Thus, never forget that struggle and when you want to return to old habits, remember how long it took you to lose weight and also remember the money you paid to get better (because no one wants to pay more money than they need to!). You don't need to go back, and you have the skills to keep moving forward.

Keep a picture of your old self handy. You can pull this picture out when you need a visual reminder of how far you've come. Remember that "old you" and know that you don't want to be them anymore. You've become a person that makes you happier, and there's no need to sabotage the better you. Respect your personal growth by loving the person you were without wanting to be that person anymore. You were fine just as you were in the past, but your changed self feels better, and that's the difference.

Remember how bad you felt before you made a change. You wanted to change for a reason! You weren't comfortable in your skin before you made the change, so you need never to forget that you changed for a reason. You wanted to grow as a person, and you accomplished this goal by dreaming of a better self and working to make that person a reality.

Think of how much better you feel now that you've made a change. Doesn't it feel exhilarating to take an issue and watch as it gradually improves? Of course, it does, so take that victorious feeling and carry it with you whenever temptation may strike. When you want to eat a whole bag of chips, think of how much better you'd feel if you didn't do that. Think of how good it will feel to choose a snack that will fuel your body with nutrients and care. Use that feeling to maintain your good habits.

Promise yourself that you're never going to go backward.

Repeat this message to yourself every day if you need to because if you tell yourself that it won't happen, your brain is likely to listen. You have to keep going forward, or you'll end up running in dissatisfying circles. It can be so easy to get stuck in the past and let everything that allured you into a false sense of security, but by relying so much on the past, you will lose sight of the present, and you will forfeit much of the happiness you could have by not seeing all the beautiful things that are right there in front of you.

Know that the future is yours for the taking. You decide what you want your future to be, and you build it. There are some variables in life that you have no power over, and those things can be terrifying and make you not want to think about the future.

You get hurt, people die, you change jobs, etc. Lots of things will change in the future in ways you can't predict, but you have the power to take those changes positively or negatively. Any change can be used to better yourself in some way. You just have to determine how you will use that change to your advantage.

Choose healthy choices. Once you've lost weight, you are not going to stop eating nutrient-dense foods. Your body still needs fruits, vegetables, healthy fats, proteins, and whole grains just as much as it did before. Don't start turning to foods with empty calories for meals.

Continue to cook well-balanced meals and eat foods that are good for your body, and that will give you the energy you need to carry you through the day.

Always tend to your emotional and physical needs. These needs should come before anything else. Prioritize what your body wants from you and let your body be cherished instead of degraded. Continue to practice mindful eating and remain aware of your emotions to ensure that you don't neglect your body or mind.

You've worked so hard to make progress, so it would make you feel like the worst person alive to go back on those changes once you've finally reached your weight loss goal. Accordingly, you need to keep reminding yourself of how far you've come so that the victory of your weight loss is always fresh in your mind. Feel proud of your progress, proud enough that you hold yourself accountable to keep up that progress even when it is hard to do so (because some days will be harder than others).

STAY ACTIVE

Humans need activity. It's important to keep doing things and accomplishing physical feats even if you've already met your goal weight. Once you've lost weight, you may be able to ease up on the intense physical activity, but it will hurt your physical and emotional health to quit being active altogether.

Boredom is one of the biggest reasons people overeat, so keep yourself busy to avoid the pitfalls of having nothing to do but eat as you watch TV.

Continue your physical activity. If you've found physical activities that you love, don't quit once you've reached your goal weight. Continue to let them better your life and drive you to be a happier and healthier person. Stay in tune with your body's needs and find power in all the wonderful things your body can do.

Challenge the activity you already do and try to keep pushing yourself. I bet that you can be doing more than you are. Don't let your workout regime become stagnant.

Keep pushing your skills and building your body up. You should never be content with how you are right now. You can always do more and improve your physical condition.

Maintain hobbies that bring your fulfillment. Studies have shown that hobbies are good for your health and to reduce stress. These hobbies don't have to be physical, but keeping hobbies will give you purpose, and projects help keep you motivated. You need to have outlets for your creative energy, which can be found through hobbies. Your hobbies should be recreational and have nothing to do with your work or other responsibilities. Hobbies such as constructing models, writing, or drawing are all just a few ideal options for people to consider. Some of the most common hobbies are games, collecting things, outdoor activity, or building things. The possibilities are endless!

Be mentally active. Finding pursuits that challenge your brain can be a strong way to keep yourself occupied. Maybe you like to complete puzzles. Maybe you like to write stories. Maybe you like to solve riddles. Maybe you like to read books. Whatever it is that keeps your mind active, do it. Your brain is a muscle, and you can train it just as you can other parts of your body, so don't neglect your brain. It will get boring if you don't keep it on its toes!

Spend time with people who make you feel good about yourself. Maintain quality friendships once you have lost weight. Don't find people who only accept you because you have lost weight or who will make you feel bad about yourself. Choose to spend your time with people who will keep you engaged in your relationships and feeling confident about those friendships. Supportive people are just as important when you maintain your weight as when you lose weight.

Being active is one of the best ways to maintain your weight, and it doesn't matter what methods you choose to keep you busy, but try to maintain several things that keep you staying strong and reaching for opportunities that make you happy and secure in your position in life. Being active will help you keep bad habits out.

8

Emotional Eating

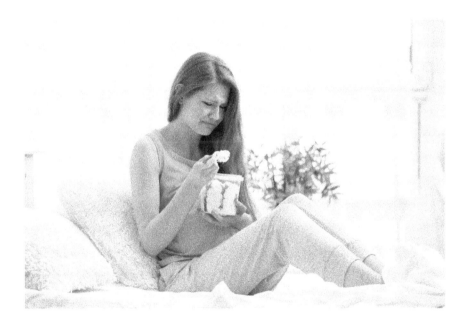

Food cravings also represent a symptom of emotional tension. We react by emotional eating that can function for a brief period but typically ends in us feeling much worse. Have you noticed when you're starving and seek to satiate that with food, that it doesn't work very well? That is because food isn't an effective way to satisfy mental hunger. To combat emotional eating, we need to build better coping mechanisms to affect our emotions, feelings, and behave differently. Below are a few observations.

Using Sensitivity to Create a Difference In Any Sort of Hunger You Feel

Do you get food cravings because the body requires calories or when you want to make sure you have enough nutrition? Whether you experience internal pressure to eat or when you need to deal with an intense appetite? To become mindful of your reasons for eating, continue listening to your emotions and feelings. Listen even to what secret convictions you have regarding yourself, "I am frail, I will never do this." Beware of how you sound before and after consuming fruits and vegetables. Tell yourself, "What type of food will be suitable?

Take Time to Pinpoint Your Rituals and Triggers

Upon waking up, will you head directly to the coffee pot? Speed your way to work and stop at a bakery that offers your dream treat? Know whether you eat when you're sleepy, hungry, frustrated, etc. If you don't know when food is activated, consider rapid journaling. If you're getting shocked, note down what happened before the sensation. In the end, you may see a similar thread. Our understanding of our behaviors and causes gives us the information we need to develop new strategies for coping.

Most individuals claim they have absolutely no room for a safe lifestyle. Particularly many women struggle with this problem because they may have a deep conviction than to take care of themselves before others is selfish. I encourage you to accept the notion that self-care is not selfish. Your cup needs to be full in a safe way. Everything you're offering is in excess. Holding yourself up helps you take control of others. It lets you set a good example for your family and others around you. "When you've developed a safe, fulfilling friendship with yourself, you've got something worth sharing with others."

Make a List of Emotional-Eating Alternatives

Identify the causes, write down what you have typically done in response to them in the past, and then come up with at least three ways to adapt to the triggers in a way that promotes well-being. Examples include walking, contacting a relative, eating healthy stuff, meditating, and so on. Hold yourself on this line of thinking. We may not be able to remember such self-nurturing options when we are anxious. Also, if you don't think they can perform, test them out before you decide to eat.

Set Limitations

Make a list of which food is a "yeah," which is "maybe, at times," and which is a "no." I recommend that borders be made clear, stable, scalable, and conscious. This is particularly helpful when you experience pressure from society to consume unhealthy food. Respect your own rules, and you may see people following them too. We, as individuals, tend to live up to our expectations because we don't have to dread having them. You do not need permission or recognition from others. Inside you, you will build a foundation of protection that another individual does not need to give and that no one else can take away. Check-in with yourself when considering a difficult decision.

Hear Your Ego or the Best Self

Play the judgment options out to the limit of your head and check in with how you feel at the moment. Be responsible for your emotions.

No matter what happens, inside of you, the response is decided. When you accuse someone else of you are being disempowered from finding solutions.

Be In Attendance

It empowers you to live with the current body option and not linger in the past or predict what's going to happen in the future—using perceived failures of the past as learning experiences. Don't let the potential mold the past. Any new experience represents an opportunity to make new choices. If you're off-line, just start over again. The emotions that drive you to consume have a meaning that you need to get across to you.

Listen and consider what they have to tell so you won't have to repress them. Then you can let them go. Instead of listening to your thoughts, you will react. Remember always that all the experiences are impermanent.

To Savor the Joy of Eating

Most eating is performed habitually without knowledge. Look out for the light, the scent, the touch, the sound, and the taste of food. Have you ever got to the end of a meal and realize that you didn't know how it tasted? Do you get more because you want to try it? Eat with attention from the outset. Recognize the difference between "complete" and "not hungry any longer" Get over the idea of cleaning your plate; just eat until you feel full.

Tell yourself, is my lifestyle/environment enabling my goal to manifest itself? Do you have all the necessary cooking supplies to prepare healthy meals? Did you remove temptations from your household? Should you spend time with those individuals who inspire you? What restaurants do you want to eat at? Do you go out to meet a friend for a meal or a stroll in the park? Do you talk about the things you're aspiring to and interested in, or what you're worried about, or what you don't like?

How often in our minds do we fail to watch ourselves? And then our mistakes keep repeating?

Refocus Your Feelings

Replace the "I can't have that" feeling with "I want something else"

Focus your attention on wealth and appreciate what you do, instead of dwelling on weakness or loss. And note, starting to like new things.

Define Your Feelings

Will you view the "I just eat something terrible" feeling as "I'm a bad person" or "I won't be able to do this?" React to these thoughts in the way a friend would. Use kind and caring expressions. This could contradict those thoughts: "I made a decision that was not in my best interest. That is not to say that I am a failure or that I cannot make healthy decisions. Just now, I feel that way because I've already made a wrong decision, but every moment is another excellent opportunity to make a different choice. So far, at this moment, I will be present and make the right decision. Eat well!

Pay attention to how comfortable you feel and how much you love the sensation as you make the right decision. To get you going, keep a journal of your achievements. You can't force trust, or bravery, or patience, but you can plant it, nurture it, and evolve with it.

Affirmations are a tool to nourish yourself. In the present tense, affirmations are positive statements designed to train one's consciousness in a constructive direction.

"Repeating an assertion brings the subconscious to that state of consciousness in which it acknowledges what it wants to believe."

Lastly, I invite you to consider the possibility of you being able to have health. Was it something you accepted? Were you clinging to that negative image of yourself?

Are you able to let go of those feelings or identity? Will you owe yourself permission to remain healthy?

Psychology and Common Causes of Emotional Eating

When we improve on the types of foods we consume, we will most likely be able to control certain involuntary impulses and cravings and manage our weight better. Did you know the way your day plays out is determined by what you eat? You really are what you eat. That's not just a cliché. It's true.

When you do not eat enough or you consume too much food, it can seriously affect your health and your way of life. This might paint a morbid image of food in your mind, but don't let it. Remember, balance is key. That's why people are less likely to eat foods that have caused them to vomit. A person is less likely to retry the food for fear of repeating the experience.

Emotional eating is, to some extent, physiological. When we are stressed, our bodies have an activation of the sympathetic nervous system or a "fight or flight" reaction.

A rush of adrenaline is part of the fight or flight response. We need energy to "survive" stress. When we consume calories while food is metabolized, a signal is sent to the brain that the body has enough energy to run or fight, and our brain "turns off" the sympathetic response.

After a few bites, our bodies feel safe and go into a state of the parasympathetic nervous system, which slows us down, relaxes us, and gives us comfort. In other words, it works! But it works until it does. This is where consciousness comes into play.

Emotional eating behaviors often stem from influences from early life, like the influence of parents' and caregivers' eating habits, the foods used as a reward or punishment, programs that guide eating habits, colleagues, diets, and rules. They can all influence eating later in life. However, early and current dietary influences are rarely based on hunger.

Babies know that they can stop breastfeeding or drinking from a bottle when they are full - their bodies are tuned to the signs of hunger and satisfaction. They are the perfect conscious eaters. Later, the variety of external dietary influences disconnects the body from these intrinsic internal stimuli.

Who's the Boss? Your Head or Your Stomach?

You have to be in control of your body and your mind. You have to be the dominant character when making food choices and not your feelings. When you are in control, you are more likely to make an effort to cut back on foods you know present a serious risk to your health.

If you leave your feelings in charge, you will end up eating what feels good and kills you slowly. You'll wind up like a huge whale with a ticking time bomb in it.

While we always have it at the back of our minds to eat healthy, stay hydrated, and sleep well, all this is often easier said than done. It's like a very vivid dream you have and then forget when you wake up. Keep in mind the keyword here is will. Will! As in the driving need to fulfill a set goal.

Psychology and Emotional Eating

You might wonder what psychology has to do with emotional eating. Well, psychology studies human behavior. It studies why humans act the way they do. For people trying to find a way to manage emotional eating, psychology will help. How?

It addresses your character. Your eating behaviors and patterns would need to be observed, so an action plan tailored to your needs can be designed.

You can identify your thought patterns. Your thoughts and emotions would need to be analyzed. You can then discover what your emotional triggers are. Once your cognitive pattern has been thoroughly explored with the help of a licensed professional, they can then figure out a fitting solution to the problem.

The truth is no matter what solutions are proffered, they just won't work unless you're ready to make a change. You have to be willing to drop emotional eating and lead a healthier life. Your decision must be unwavering. This requires putting a lot of effort into achieving success, limiting distractions, and setting targets.

You also have to be self-aware. Become mindful. Do not act unconsciously. Just observe and watch for triggers that induce specific cravings. Then, be careful of what you eat and how much you do it.

Try replacing your sugary confections with something sugary but healthy, like an apple or pineapple. Whenever you start to have your cravings for a pastry, try to replace it with something healthier. It won't be easy, but where there's a will, there's a way. How do you get the will? Find your why. When you have solid, concrete reasons for wanting to make a change, you'll find the "how" gets that much more achievable.

There is nothing more satisfying than looking back at some mistakes you have made and seeing that you have overcome them. Yes, the past may have shaped your undesirable present. But the present shapes the future; every moment you spend wallowing in self-pity, body shaming yourself, and languishing in the throes of a broken heart just keeps you from achieving the final goal.

If you stick with me, I'm going to give you the tools you need to overcome your emotional eating. You just have to decide that you can, and you will. Against all odds. It's no secret people tend to get what they want if they put their all into it.

So, are you with me? I want you all in. Whenever you want to quit, I want you to remember why you started. I want you to know I'm rooting for you. I want you to know I've seen countless people beat emotional eating. I've seen it happen, so I know it can be done. I know you can do it. But I can only hold your hand. You're going to have to put one foot in front of the other and take this journey with me. Can you do it? Will you do it?

Are you worth it?

Don't turn the page until you realize and feel deeply in your bones the only correct answer to that question.

Yes. You are worth it. So very worth it.

Eating Disorders

BINGE EATING

Food can start to become scary. How much you desire it is so challenging. Why does it taste so good to eat a loaf of bread? The amount of relief that comes along when you can hold an entire gallon of ice cream and eat it directly with a spoon is like the same comfort a warm blanket can bring.

Binge eating can be defined as any period of time that is spent eating an excess of food. People will often binge unhealthy foods at first, though those in recovery might find that they end up binging "healthy" things like vegetables, tea, and water. It is a pattern of stuffing yourself to the point where you feel both physically and mentally ill. These periods are usually done alone and always involve a level of shame and embarrassment.

Binging isn't enjoyable, or at least isn't the entire time. At first, there's the satisfaction of the taste, texture, and security in the amount of food you're consuming.

Then, by the fourth or fifth burger, or taco, or a slice of pizza, it starts to set in that you shouldn't be doing that and that you can stop at any moment. But we keep eating, hoping to numb that logical voice in our heads.

A recorded 3 to 5% of women and 2% of men suffer from a binge eating disorder. However, many more go undiagnosed because of the stigma that surrounds eating disorders. Those who have never suffered from an eating disorder won't be the most understanding about it, either. When you have bulimia, people might recognize that you are doing something unhealthy, and this is when people start to get serious. Throwing up over and over again can mess up your body on the inside, destroying your throat and liver. Anorexia and binge eating are dangerous as well, but people won't always initially see these as dangerous acts, especially if you are over or underweight.

Those who are underweight that binge eat don't seem like they have a problem. Some people might even look at you and make comments like, "you should gain weight," or "you are all skin and bones!" The same goes for those who are overweight and anorexic. If you go through periods of starvation as a person that's 275 pounds, people aren't going to be as concerned. Some might even encourage this behavior.

Those statistics make up almost 1 out of 20 people you will meet, and yet we still have so many confused ideologies around binge eating, overeating, anorexia, and bulimia.

Many people with binge eating disorders might develop anorexia or bulimia in response to the binge periods, or they might have had them first, which led to the binging. Either way, both are very unhealthy and can cause a person to live in shame and agony that only makes their condition worse. We do unhealthy things and then try to do things we think are healthy to remedy them. But these are still unhealthy things. Those who suffer from anorexia and bulimia might do this because they think it is better for their bodies, as a way to respond to the overeating they put it through, first. In reality, though, it's just another unhealthy coping mechanism.

BULIMIA

Bulimia will usually start with periods of binging, though some people can develop bulimia without having a binge disorder first. Most diagnostics do involve individuals who go through binges of food that are much larger than what the average person would eat. Bulimia is a response to make up for this binge, usually resulting in people purging themselves of the food they just ate.

Bulimia isn't just throwing up. Many people will buy laxatives and take them right after they binged in order to help move things through their bodies quickly enough that they don't gain weight. Bulimia will cause your body to lose weight, but in the process, it is an unhealthy habit that destroys many other parts of your body. First and foremost, it puts a lot of stress on your body and mind. Those who are bulimic are silent sufferers, keeping their actions hidden from other people.

It can also be very dangerous to your heart. Some people who are bulimic will even suffer a heart attack, though they may be dangerously underweight because our hearts weren't designed to take on unnecessary laxatives or the stress of throwing up on a regular basis. It can also result in stomach and intestinal issues, such as inflammation, gastric reflux, and gastroparesis, which is when your stomach muscles become partially paralyzed.

Some people might think you're doing it for attention. I've known individuals who have said their parents or siblings told them they just wanted attention when they were throwing up, especially those who weren't obviously underweight. People might think you can't be bulimic if you are not a size 0 with obvious bone shadows in your body or a gaunt-looking face. This disease is anything but an attempt at attention.

Excuses become a regular thing. You'll especially hear excuses from those who participate in athletic activities. Wrestlers trying to gain weight will simply say they're only doing it while they wait to weigh in. Those who participate in beauty competitions or even brides about to get married will say they're just doing it until they can fit into a dress.

People will say they're just trying to lose twenty pounds, and then they'll stop. These are all excuses, and many people who are bulimic have said them before.

There is so much shame involved in the process. Bulimia usually comes in response to a mental illness, such as anxiety or depression. If there isn't one initially, one will likely develop. It is a process of hiding the binge period, and then the purge time, as well. Sometimes, these have to be separate occurrences, though there is anxiety to purge soon after binging. You might binge eat in your car while on break at work, and then you have to make it to the bathroom fast before your body starts actually to digest the food as it should. On the way into work, however, a coworker might stop and chat—but the entire time, your heart will be racing, hoping you can make it to the bathroom in time to throw up your big lunch.

How to Stop Emotional Eating

Some of us have participated in emotional eating for some point or another. Emotional eating occurs if we eat to soothe wounded feelings or cope with a stressful situation. Emotional eating can occur after a hard day at work, a fight with a loved one, or when the kids run around the house crying. The first step to avoiding emotional eating is to become conscious that it is occurring.

In the course of the day, ask yourself many times how you feel to stop a significant amount of tension. Recognize the symptoms of discomfort or tension. Find a way to convey the feelings efficiently so they can be published. Holding in negative or hurtful feelings may lead to a binge later on. Stopping to evaluate your emotions during the day can also help you pause before reaching for unhealthy foods.

Second, preventing causes. Think back to the last emotional eating moment. What happened just before you would eat? Remember not being hungry and feeding anyway? Do you still eat after a difficult job meeting or dispute with a co-worker? Identifying and preventing emotional-eating activities can help deter potential occurrences.

Third, try doing something else while eating happens.

By monitoring your emotional state during the day, you will be conscious of when emotional eating will occur and seeking solutions to it.

When eating fattening foods makes you feel confident and relaxed, build a list of other habits contributing to the same feelings. Exercise is an important way to promote positive feelings. Other suggestions are hot baths, reading a good book, or watching your favorite movie.

Keep the activity list on your refrigerator to remind you of alternative suggestions should a deficiency occur. Journaling is another way to avoid emotional eating.

Tracking feelings, anxieties, fears, and emotions will help you recognize causes. After keeping a list for a few days, look back for specific feelings that made you emotionally eat. Recurring things like job stress that require action to alleviate tension or situations that make you feel stressed. Another strategy to reduce emotional eating is to cut your portions in half. If you have had a busy day and have a meal, place half-sized portions on your plate and assess how you feel after you have eaten. If you are still hungry, you might eat more, but if you are feeling depressed and looking for warmth, take a moment to consider your motives. Assessing your appetite and emotional state will avoid overeating. Stop comforts like white bread and processed sugars.

These foods actually cover negative emotions and cannot satisfy you until the meal is finished. You need to drink plenty of water during your meal. Recognize when you are complete and stop.

Finally, if you emotionally eat, forgive yourself. If you keep thinking negatively about yourself, you are just accepting more tension and the opportunity to eat emotionally. Bad eating habits take years to establish and are uncorrectable overnight. Work for small goals and reward yourself when you enjoy something other than food.

Weight Loss Hypnosis and Controlling Emotional Eating Behaviors

TRAUMA AND STRESS

When a certain type of trauma or stress occurs in your life, many people gain weight. Divorce, death, and even unstable families and friends make many people feel relaxed when eating. Also, after stress, your emotional eating patterns are in place, and your relaxation is a natural pattern for you. One of the main goals of hypnosis for weight loss is to retrain the brain to overcome these ingrained behaviors.

EMOTIONAL HUNGER

This emotional appetite is not just due to stress and trauma. Emotional hunger also comes from adolescence, events that arise with peers and learned behavior. Most overweight people eat to relieve the pain or fill a hole in life.

It feels so good to eat, and sometimes you feel guided by food when everything else is out of control. Hypnosis in weight loss aims to remove these mental causes so that you do not consume foods.

TRUE PHYSICAL HUNGER

Many people have forgotten what real physical hunger is due to emotional eating habits. When you clear your mind of these negative learned habits, it is easy to know when you are hungry. It is a slow phase, and true hunger does not just strike you out of the blue. You can feel lightheaded and lethargic when your stomach starts rumbling; this is because your brain is signaling that it is hungry. If you get these signals, it means that the time has come to eat and avoid starvation. However, true hunger is hard to recognize from emotional stimuli. So it is important to turn to a method that will help you quickly!

WEIGHT LOSS HYPNOSIS COULD BE THE KEY

Hypnosis for weight loss is an effective treatment that can help you to eradicate mental deprivation and emotional eating patterns for good from your life. You can go beyond computational models that have held you back for many years by simply getting into a relaxed state and listening to audio files that help you reframe your thought. Would it not be nice to reprogram your mind and body in another way to manage stress and emotional eating?

Wouldn't it feel wonderful if you could act differently seamlessly so that you can really accomplish your objectives?

The Causes of Emotional Eating

Emotional eating is often associated with eating as a response to emotions. The emotions could be positive or negative, but in most cases, it happens when your external struggles start affecting your internal dialogue. This leaves you feeling overwhelmed and creates a negative emotional state, and as a result of it, you start eating your emotions.

Emotional eating is not about food, and your physical hunger does not drive it. It is driven by seeking comfort.

The eating habits of an emotional eater are often driven by his or her unfulfilled needs, which are accompanied by the strong emotions of shame, anxiety, sadness, stress, anger, frustration, *etc.* People often get overwhelmed with these emotions, and they try to control them with food, not always realizing that this will only make the situation worse. Maybe you have already noticed that using food to cope with your feelings never provides you with the much-needed comfort that you were seeking.

Emotional eating is aimed at pushing negative feelings away in order to feel better, but after eating the food for emotional reasons, you probably notice that you are still feeling dissatisfied.

Food can never remove bad feelings or fill the hole inside you. You may feel slightly better for a little while, but it is not a long-term solution.

Emotional eating usually involves choosing to eat mainly unhealthy foods, or large quantities of it, in order to feel less lonely or happier or having more control over your life. Emotional eating is also called comfort eating and is driven by your stresses, insecurities, fears, and anxieties. When you feel sad, you reach for a chocolate bar. When you feel lonely, you overeat. Negative feelings can then become triggers that lead to binging or unhealthy eating without even thinking about it. You simply do it on autopilot.

Sometimes eating this way can help, but most often, it cannot. It can create more problems than you had before. At times it gives you temporary relief and the comfort that you were searching for, but it is always—and I mean always—a short-term solution. It might provide you with a temporary feeling of pleasure, but when this feeling is gone, you are then left with nothing, so you need another fix.

It is important to understand that no amount of food will ever satisfy an emotional eater because an emotional eater is not physically hungry. An emotional eater does not always eat because of his or her physiological need—the hunger; he or she eats to suffocate feelings that they struggle to deal with.

I want to highlight something important here, and that is that we are all emotional eaters at times, and eating this way is nothing to be ashamed of. We all have moments of weakness that we try to control in different ways.

Eating certain foods when we are not feeling hungry is very much about trying to take control or get rid of certain emotions that are overwhelming us or making us feel bad. In order to start managing our eating behaviors better, it is important to understand that we are in control of our eating and not the other way around. Our eating is not in control of us unless we allow it to be.

When you are eating for any other reason apart from hunger, it does not matter how much food you eat, and it does not matter what you eat; the problem is that no amount of food will ever fill the hole inside you, and no amount of food will ever fully satisfy you. Some people choose alcohol to fill the hole, and others use drugs, but the majority of people choose food. Remember that when you want to eat because you are upset or stressed, the food is probably not what you need at that moment. Think of the most loving thing you can give to yourself when you want food, and make sure you get it. Understanding that there is an alternative to overeating and binging when you need comfort, it will put the power back into your hands.

Food is easily accessible to most people, and it is part of our everyday life. We all need to eat to live; therefore, food is the most common form of abuse, and many people find it hard to resist and control. Even though at first sight it does not seem to be too damaging for us, the food we eat can actually be extremely dangerous for our health and weight, depending on the choices we make.

Tips for Managing Stress to Avoid Emotional Eating

No matter what your binge eating cycles are like, stress is nearly bound to encourage you to act out with emotional eating.

When it involves stress and its ability to influence your dietary behaviors, there are generally two ways in which it can happen.

The first is that you simply end up feeling stressed, and you binge eat as how to make some sort of comfort in your life so that you're not feeling quite as stressed anymore. The opposite way includes you feeling so stressed that you simply think that you cannot eat, then binge eating when your body cannot take the stress-induced fasting anymore. In either scenario, stress can negatively affect your diet and may also become a negative coping method that worsens your binge eating in the future, too.

Furthermore, both of those behavioral patterns around stress and eating can cause weight gain, which suggests that they're not productive to your goals of weight loss.

Managing stress to avoid emotional eating largely revolves around you learning the way to deal with and manage your stress properly. The more proactive you'll be in handling your pressure, the less likely you're to hunt out behaviors like binge eating as a chance to assist you to overcome the strain that you simply are experiencing.

People who routinely experience problematic binge eating, thanks to stress or other emotions, will often use practices like meditating, preventative self-care, and routine relaxationpractices to assist them in reducing stress.

This way, they're less likely to interact with emotional eating in the first place.

When it involves handling bursts of upper-stress levels, meditating is often incredibly helpful in assisting you with bringing your stress levels to backtrack. This way, you're more likely to feel asleep and less susceptible to feel the necessity to affect your stress through less healthy means, like through overeating.

Preventative self-care measures that will assist you in affecting your stress are incredibly useful in avoiding stress in the first place.

For instance, budgeting more effectively so that you're not so worried about money, creating a bank account, exercising daily, and spending time with loved ones are all great ways to avoid scenarios where your stress may rise unnecessarily.

The simpler you're at handling areas of your life that typically end in stress, the simpler you'll be in eliminating your stress. Or, when it can't be removed, you can minimize it so you feel more in control of your life.

Routine relaxation practices are almost like preventative self-care, except that they're more focused on the day to day practices that are meant to assist you to relax regardless of what has triggered your stress.

For example, some people relax after a work-day by gardening, reading a book, or just resting on the couch with their eyes closed so that they take time to decompress from the day they had. Some people chose to take a candlelit bath, go for a walk, or maybe play a game on their laptop as a way to destress. The thought here is that you find a simple but good way to decompress whenever you are feeling stressed, that you can do on a day to day basis so that your stress doesn't begin to rise an excessive amount.

When you want to manage your stress to avoid overeating, the simplest thing you'll do is try new routines and rituals until you discover practices that assist you in destressing without overeating.

The exact "formula" for destressing is going to be different for everybody, so you're going to need to take a moment to seek out that information for yourself.

The higher you understand your own needs around stress and the ways to relax, the more likely you're to be ready to come up with a practice that can assist you in destressing in the first place.

The Cycle of Emotional Eating

To overcome emotional eating, you need to identify the triggers.

Emotional eating always starts with one or more triggers. These triggers often include positive or negative feelings. Negative feelings are more common, and when we experience them, we try to use food to cope with them. The problem is that the food can never solve emotional problems.

We looked at the diet cycle. Now we are going to look at the cycle of emotional eating, what it is, and how it can affect you:

Step 1: the emotional eating cycle starts with a trigger. It is always caused by one or more triggers. Emotions associated with triggers could be any of the following: rejection, sadness, boredom, frustration, anxiety, emptiness, loneliness, and many more. Whatever the trigger is, it is often an emotion that you struggle with and want to suppress.

Step 2: is the need for comfort and choosing to eat the food you love in order to make yourself feel better.

The foods you choose to eat often tend to be unhealthy, high in sugar, and contain lots of salt and trans fats. Some of these foods often include pizzas, chocolates, cakes, and sugary soft drinks, which could be very damaging to your health as well.

Step 3: provokes feelings of relief and finally feeling good. This good feeling does not last long, but it is a solution to your problem when you need it the most.

Step 4: positive feelings leave you. Then you step into the feeling-sorry-for-yourself zone. You are feeling sad or angry at yourself for eating the food you just had.

The cycle finishes with experiencing feelings of guilt, blame, and/or disappointment. You regret the way you acted. You are angry at yourself because you ate all those unhealthy foods. You feel upset about your behavior, and you need some comfort. So, once again, you turn to food, as this creates good feelings for you.

And then the cycle repeats itself again. You are back to step 1, then step 2, then 3, then 4, and after completing step 5, you start all over again.

Being stuck in the cycle of emotional eating can lead to binge eating. Binge eating is created by the desire to improve your mood and to feel better and is associated with uncontrollably eating large quantities of food each time you binge. This can cause physical and psychological discomfort and can result in feeling unhappy or bad about yourself, and it often causes further binging and more unhappiness. And in order to feel better, you may binge eat again.

It is a vicious cycle—feeling bad, then overeating, then feeling bad because of overeating, then binging in order to feel better—and it carries on.

Eating because of your emotions is a coping mechanism that is not removing physical hunger. The focus is to find a way to make your feelings go away.

Eating Your Emotions

How often do you feel very hungry? How often do you feel so hungry that it does not matter what you eat; you would be happy with it? Not very often, I believe. In this day and age, not many people allow themselves to get too hungry. They tend to eat before they ever get hungry.

Eating unhealthily, or in some cases, simply the act of eating is often caused by the triggers associated with emotional fulfillment. We all have different ways of dealing with feelings of fulfillment, but sometimes we respond to it by eating our emotions and looking for comfort in food, hoping that the emotions will go away with each bite we take.

A chocolate bar can never cure loneliness, and cake cannot permanently remove anxiety. Short-term relief is the best we can hope for.

Trying to suppress emotions that bring discomfort and turning to food instead will not bring the desired outcome. To make your stress, sadness, anger, anxiety, or frustration go away, you need to explore where they are coming from and what the cause is, and find ways to deal with them appropriately.

When something is present but hidden under the layers, it is far away from your reach, and you may find it too hard to understand its meaning. Finding a way to understand your emotions will help you create a better connection with yourself.

Emotional eating is often driven by the desire to hide, to cover, or to replace the negative feelings that you might be experiencing. As described before, when stuck in the cycle of emotional eating, feeling guilty, disappointed, ashamed, or angry with yourself is very common.

This can then lead to beating yourself up and giving yourself a hard time for not being able to manage your behavior better.

Common Causes of Emotional Eating

STRESS

Have you ever noticed that stress makes you hungry?

Then you're not alone. When stress is chronic, our bodies tend to produce high levels of cortisol (the stress hormone).

Cortisol evokes the need for sweet and fried foods and salty foods that give you lots of energy and joy. The higher the stress in your life, the more likely you are to turn to food for emotional relief.

FILL YOUR EMOTIONS

Eating can be seen as a means of temporarily silencing or "filling" unpleasant feelings, such as fear, sadness, loneliness, resentment, fear, and shame. While paralyzed by food, you can avoid the difficult feelings you prefer not to have.

BOREDOM OR FEELING EMPTY

Have you ever eaten to give yourself something to do or to fill a void in your life? You feel empty and unhappy, and food seems like a way to fill your mouth, and this time distracts you from the underlying feelings of emptiness and dissatisfaction in your life.

CHILDHOOD HABITS

It's normal for parents to reward their kid's good behavior with ice cream, get pizza if they get good grades, or sweets if they are sad. Or your food can be enlivened by fond memories of grilling hamburgers with your father or eating cookies with your mother. These habits often carry on to adulthood.

SOCIAL INFLUENCES

Eating with other people seems to be an excellent way to relieve stress, but it can also lead to overeating. It's easy to overeat simply because the food is there or because everyone eats. You can also overeat on a social occasion due to nervousness. Or maybe your family or friends encourage you to overeat.

You have probably seen yourself in at least one of the descriptions above. But if you still want to be more specific, one way to identify the patterns behind your emotional eating is to keep a journal.

When you feel compelled to overeat, take a moment to understand what is causing the urge. In this way, you will generally experience a shocking event that triggered the emotional cycle of food.

Record everything in your food diary: what did you eat, how did you feel before eating, what did you feel while eating, and what did you feel after? Over time, a pattern will emerge!

Become a Mindful Eater

These additional tips for dealing with emotional food:

Resist a moral value that creates embarrassment when eating: "good" versus "bad" food and "clean" versus "dirty" food.

Ask yourself if you are starving or eating due to stress.

Try to "control yourself." Strive to understand the different feelings of hunger during the day and meals.

Identify the different activities that relax you and what you can do to avoid eating emotionally.

Using a personal "hunger indicator" can help restore body-mind communication. It internalizes the hunger signs, making it more challenging to remove external influences. The strategy is to pay more attention to how you feel and evaluate these emotions on a scale of 0 to 10. This helps the body to perceive, understand, and be more aware of the internal sensations during food.

The hunger indicator collects data and, if the experience is good, the variables (the type of food, quality, quantity, time, etc.) can be repeated.

Otherwise, they can be edited and commented on mentally or in a journal. This approach to data collection also helps reduce food embarrassment, as we are less likely to overeat when we are aware of it, rather than making a mistake when eating.

Another strategy is to ask yourself if you are hungry or stressed. If you physically assess hunger before, during, and after eating, this can guide you on how much to eat and what to eat.

If it is emotional, discuss step by step:

What is the feeling?

Where does it come from?

Replace it with other activities that create joy and comfort.

This three-in-one relationship can help you overcome your emotional eating. Food creates joy in the brain, but many other actions can trigger pleasure. Use three more actions as a substitute to balance the pleasure of eating emotionally. This offers a break and an opportunity to control your desires.

Activities like drinking a cup of tea, having a bath, walking or listening to music, or a combination of these actions activates the parasympathetic nervous system and progressive response to relaxation and stress management.

Emotional eating is often violent and banal, as health and nutrition experts believe, this could be one of the main reasons why people are more obese than ever. We eat because we are happy or sad more than when we are starving, and the food we eat in such situations is often far from healthy. So, there is a problem because emotional eating tends to consume large amounts of unhealthy food. Obesity, diabetes, heart disease, and other health problems are the result of poor nutrition.

So, it makes a lot of sense to stop eating in response to mood or feelings, and only by eating correctly can you avoid the long list of health problems.

THE ANSWER = HYPNOSIS

Hypnosis allows us to speak directly to the subconscious mind while avoiding the conscious mind, and relaxation techniques and specific language patterns will enable you to reprogram your mental beliefs.

If successful, hypnosis has proven to be almost a miracle cure. The list of physical and mental problems that hypnosis has been able to treat effectively is varied and almost infinite.

Your unconscious mind forms new habits incredibly fast, which means that hypnotherapy can quickly cure your unhealthy episodes of emotional eating when everything else you've tried has failed.

Healthy hypnosis will begin with you lying down comfortably, closing your eyes, and trying to eliminate thoughts and emotions from the mind.

After a few sessions, you might start to notice being more in control of your emotional reactions and dealing better with anxiety and stress; Since stress is one of the primary triggers for emotional eating, hypnosis can end it once and for all!

OTHER IMPORTANT TIPS

Practicing mindfulness gives you a complete focus on the meal. And it continues to pay attention to the food you consume when you raise the pot.

A few suggestions for feeding mindfulness are as follows:

- Consciously consider which products to purchase from the grocery store. This involves determining the worth of each object on a shopping list, thinking about each transaction, to stop buying impulsively.
- Eat when the hunger is mild. When you are waiting for your stomach to grumble to eat, you reach for the most urgent incentive. To avoid gorging, feed yourself according to a timetable.
- Take a look at the cravings. Ask whether you have real hunger or are inspired by something else to feed (e.g., pain, habit, time of

day, etc.). Analyze what induces the cravings and what triggers them to fade.

- Only feed gently! This will be helpful if you use the non-dominant hand because it allows you to take your time.
- Take little bites. Position your utensils on the side of your plate as you chew and bring your attention to the food's flavors.
- Express thanks. Contemplate the measures you have taken to bring the meal to your mouth.

Note, the capacity to be conscious is a talent. Through diligent practice, it will become easier to understand the full effects and be reflective in your mindfulness practice.

9

Reprogramming Your Mind for Success

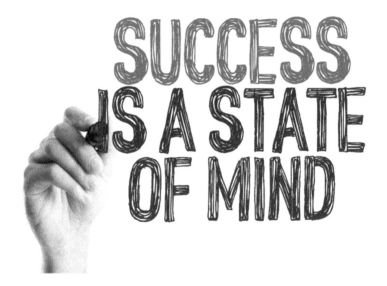

The mind is powerful. And to understand how the mind can be reprogrammed with hypnosis, we must understand the conscious and subconscious mind. The conscious mind comprises of all the waking awareness, how you read, learn, reason, everything. The subconscious mind is the invisible part of our self which works behind the scene. This subconscious mind is responsible for our behavioral aspects, how we react, how we experience things, and the key to reprogramming our mind lies with the subconscious mind.

But before understanding how to reprogram the mind with hypnosis, we must understand why we need to?

The Subconscious Mind Acts Promptly Without Any Thinking

A classic example could be cutting your fingers with a knife. The conscious mind will jump to the first aid kit, treat the wound, and move on.

Meanwhile, the subconscious mind does a lot more, from creating enzymes to create a blood clot to stop the blood flow to engaging the immune system to fight bacteria or any infection.

Another example could be a fight or flight response. When we face danger or any alarming situation, our subconscious mind triggers a fight or flight response, and based on your previous experience and existing programming of the mind; you would react.

Hence, to divert the subconscious mind towards a positive direction, you need to tap into your subconscious mind.

The Subconscious Mind Is Programmed as a Child

Most of the programming happened when you are a kid. Our definitions of morality, our acceptance, our construct of family, and friends are fundamentals that you programmed as a kid.

For instance, if you were bullied throughout high school or always rejected by people around you, in the playground, at home, when someone approaches you with kindness, you would have a hard time believing it, and your subconscious mind will tell you not to believe it.

Conversely, the reverse is also true; if you have good experiences, your subconscious will guide you to be more open to such acts. Nonetheless, it is important to know neither such experience nor the programming is permanent. As a child, our mind was more open to programming, but even as an adult, our mind is still programmable. And if every time we are exposed to something good, our subconscious mind renders a flight response and unknowingly sabotages whatever good could have happened, there is a need to change yourself at the core level, at the subconscious mind level.

Survival Instinct of the Subconscious Mind

The prime objective of the subconscious mind is survival. And owing to this, there are situations where we fall prey to the whims of the subconscious mind. For instance, phobias are often regarded as deep-seated fear. Some may be afraid of closed space, some of the water or high altitude, etc. The way we act when faced with our phobic fears may not be rational, but our subconscious mind keeps you in an alarming state.

Another instance is some conditional fear like when you are performing on stage or doing public speaking. The rational self will tell you it is alright, yet the subconscious mind will not let you be at ease.

The deep-seated fear of not achieving your goal, the idea of you failing keeps popping up. The tussle between the subconscious and conscious mind continues, and seldom you can reason it out.

It requires a deeper approach, one that works at the very base from where such responses originate—to reprogram the unconscious mind. This is also important to benefit from hypnosis for weight loss.

Hypnosis helps tap into this subconscious state and helps to make changes that eventually can solve all our issues. By tapping into the hypnotic state, the conscious critical faculty of the brain is bypassed. You can then safely reprogram the subconscious brain with more affirmative, assuring suggestions from making behavioral changes to dietary changes.

This reprogramming works on the principle of neuroplasticity, which suggests that the brain's biology can be changed. With the repetition of imagery, thoughts, verbal cues, emotions, the reprogramming is achieved with time. There is no absolute proof of the change, but you sure can feel it in day to day activities and the way you react now to situations compared to the past.

Here, we will explore the practices of hypnosis to reprogram your mind for weight loss.

FIND THE RIGHT MOTIVATION TO START LOSING WEIGHT

In the practice of hypnosis, a lot has been dependent on the inner quest. The subconscious mind, which does not listen to reason and pretty much drives the show for your actions and progress, requires some motivation to cling on to.

So, before entering into the practice, let me ask you a few of the basic questions related to your weight loss journey so far.

Why do you want to shed those extra pounds?

- To be in better shape and health
- To avoid any issues with overeating
- To cure your back, starting with reducing your weight
- To avoid any complication for any medical/surgical procedure
- To pick a healthy lifestyle
- To become more acceptable in society
- To impress someone with your looks
- To find your social standings by matching with how society wants to see you
- To fit into the superficial definition of beauty, how the world defines beauty?

It is important to have your reasons right. The first 5 picks suggest reason which is more confined to self, which is driven out of need but not self-loathing or self-pity.

The latter ones are more superficial in nature, and one should not strive to change for others but only for oneself. The motivation factor will vary from person to person and age to age.

Once we have established why we want to embark on a weight loss program, let's focus on a goal, an achievable goal. Not too easy and not too far-fetched but within grasp with some effort.

FINDING INNER SERENITY

Finding inner serenity is not as much a task, but it is a practice. The more your practice peace, the more it starts to come naturally to you. You may fail in keeping it, but you should try repeatedly.

You can start by asking a few of the basic questions below:

- How much are you at peace with your life?
- How you wake up daily—with a gentle beaming smile or a heavy head?
- Do you look forward to the things the day has in store or dread it?
- Do you sleep in a regular sleep cycle or often indulge in late nights?
- Do you eat regularly or often skip breakfasts?
- How do you feel doing the daily chores and activities—happy or burdened?
- Do you indulge in excessive use of any substance abuse, alcohol, etc.?
- Do you feel that you are held back by some compulsion every time you try to change?
- Do you have any control mechanisms?
- How much are you at peace with your thoughts?
- Do you feel sometimes bogged down by incessant thoughts and cannot get rid of them?
- Do you feel the need to have the calmness to deal with your thoughts?
- How do you feel when you try to focus on something—centered or being dragged to distant corners?
- How do you feel when you are in the middle of a heated conversation?

- Do you get angry often?
- How do you feel once the pang of anger waves away?
- How do you feel when things are not going your way—aghast and miserable or need to have more patience?
- How do you feel about flattery—swayed away or gently stepping aside by acknowledging it with gratitude?
- Are you able to focus on one task at a time?
- Are you able to hold and sustain the focus for a longer or considerable period of time?
- How much are you in peace with your senses?
- How do you feel about the commitments you make to yourself—obliged to fulfill or fine to delay?
- How often do you plan your diet—often or never?
- Do you stick to your diet or eat without a sense of it?
- How do you feel about your habits—urgency, and need for change or content?
- Do you plan to do yoga & exercise and meet your plans often?
- How do you act in a matter of urgency—resorting to haste and impulse or keeping your cool and responding with sense?
- How do you feel when things are not going your way—too anxious or in peace?

I would recommend using a pen and paper to scribe the answers on a sheet of paper. This will help you analyze how your inner serenity is mapped. I would strongly urge you to answer the above questions honestly, without any sense of judgment or failure or achievement.

We can make sense of most of the questions above—the right expects answers, and with it the right form of ourselves we want to be. So, even if we are feeling anxious, and we are behaving in negative manners, it is all right. Even if we are doing everything right and have the required inner serenity, it is all right; let's not jump in triumph or loss. The idea here is to just access so that we can take the necessary steps to move toward that desired peace or maintain it.

Once we answer the questions above, we can have a better idea of where we stand and can work accordingly towards the common goal of reprogramming our mind to the appropriate levels for effective weight loss results.

FIND THE RIGHT PSYCHOLOGICAL APPROACH

Another piece of reprogramming for the brain to understand is how hypnosis affects us psychologically speaking; there are mainly three theories to describe hypnosis—The Role Theory, The Altered State Theory, and Dissociation Theory.

Role theory suggests that the person is never truly in a hypnosis kind of state, the one we call the altered consciousness. It also reflects that the person may just be acting the role of a person who is in such a state.

On the contrary, at the opposite end of the spectrum, another theory, the Altered-state theory, describes hypnosis as something which, in reality, takes you to an altered state. It confirms that the person is actually hypnotized and feels what we call as the state of hypnosis or altered consciousness.

The dissociation theory of hypnosis defines this state, where we actively dissociate our consciousness.

Here, we are putting our conscious mind at rest and leave things to our subconscious mind. Dissociation theory suggests that we split consciousness and have increased concentration and focus.

Which theory holds true is a matter of debate, but it can be established that hypnosis is effective and has the below three components—Absorption, Dissociation, and Suggestion.

Absorption

The Absorption component is the state defined by how much you are immersed in the practice of hypnosis. It is also regulated by your behavioral trait of how suggestive you are.

The more suggestive you are, the more invested you will be in the practice of hypnosis. The more invested you are in practice, the more absorbed you will feel in the state of hypnosis.

Dissociation

Dissociation is about the dissociation of awareness. It is a behavioral component. The individual is separated from the normal state of being, awareness and retains basic recognition and reflexes.

Suggestion

Lastly, the suggestion component is guiding the mind to a single idea. This component generally requires some form of guidance—usually conducted by a psychiatrist or hypnotist. Firstly, using absorption and dissociation, an individual achieves the state of trance in which all consciousness is put to rest, and we are more and more absorbed, opening our subconscious mind through suggestions. Here, a practitioner uses suggestions to unearth the feelings, behavioral component, thoughts, etc. and can lay the foundation for any kind of change.

Hence, after understanding the psychology of hypnosis, we use it to further good effect. And developing on this understating, the discipline has evolved into several therapeutic uses. It may impact one person differently from another.

It may happen at a different speed, but it is an effective tool for pain relief management, stress, anxiety or treatment for trauma, fighting fears and phobias, weight loss and weight maintenance program, etc.

Mind Tricks

The mind is a delicate matter. It can trick you into believing something and also can trick you into not believing something. To understand the human mind, we can look at a few of the existing theories to understand the conscious and unconscious mind.

As defined by Sigmund Freud, the human is comprised of ID, the superego, and the ego. The ID shows you what you want without any social norms, any changes in moral values.

A common example is seeing a thing of value or someone you are attracted to and are willing to just take it. The superego is an entirely opposite part of your personality and goes with your moral standing and stops your ID from making any harsh decisions.

There is always a constant battle between the ID and the superego, and whichever side is stronger, your personality may slide to that side. The ego is another part of your personality which balances the ID and the superego.

It rationalizes the decision-making process striking a balance. It is also the component that can be termed as "self."

Together, the ID, the superego, and the ego form the unconscious mind. Furthermore, to understand what the mind believes and how hypnosis fits into it, we can look at the below points:

THE BRAIN RELIES ON HEURISTICS

One of the ways the brain operates is that it relies on heuristics, which we have tackled in the past to limit the decision-making process. The brain takes shortcuts based on past experiences to give you a way out of any laborious exercise. Though it is an essential part of our survival by making faster decisions and also often the right decisions, this can also restrict us in believing something new and may result in mistakes.

The reason being the brain can be lazy. It wants to excessively rely on heuristics rendering your capacity to change to low.

One of the most common examples is the fear of flight. The statistics suggest it is safer than road travel and airplane travel has a lower chance of accidents occurring. But since your brain relies on the shortcut known as availability heuristic and keeps you reeling in this irrational fear of flying, you are scared.

Hypnosis can prove effective to bypass such heuristics and help you take control of your mind.

You need to reprogram your mind to get past the heuristics. And, with hypnosis, this can be achieved.

MIND AND BIAS

The mind has several kinds of cognitive biases.

These are basically predispositions that guide your decision-making process. The most common types of bias include the halo effect, the hindsight bias, and the confirmation bias.

HALO EFFECT

It is the cognitive bias that suggests how a person would be based on single traits? Generally, it takes physical appearance and assumes that if a person is good looking, that person will also be smart and intelligent. Vice versa, if you are not good-looking, you might be dull, which is also a reflection of your personality. It takes comfort in what is beautiful and rejects what is not. Hence this is also referred to as the "Physical Attractiveness Stereotype."

Bypassing such a bias is important in making the right decisions. To not simply reject something based on a single trait and superficial appearance, which our mind will be so inclined to do.

THE HINDSIGHT BIAS

It is the bias where we confirm the prediction of a future event without even knowing the actual output.

Casually remarked as the "I-knew-it-all-along" phenomenon, the hindsight bias reinforces that the output of the event was known all along.

This may be comforting for some as it motivates people to know that the world outside is not random but predictable. It helps them make finance or healthcare decisions. However, it can also restrict you from making the right decision as well, especially when we are talking about something new. Hypnosis can help to open our minds to overcome such a bias and motivate us better to stick to say the weight loss program and not act rashly and give up.

THE CONFIRMATION BIAS

Takes the data into account and molds it in a fashion to meet with your existing beliefs. Here, you operate entirely just to make whatever you already believe as the only truth. You may shut your objectivity, only look at the data that fits and ignore the portions, or even not remember the data which is against your belief.

A common example can be seen in someone's orientation of a political party or a football club. If that person is a die-hard supporter of a club or party, you will find that how they navigate through the information and choose only those that confirm and that suits their purpose to expand their existing belief.

One of the challenges of the practitioner is to open the mind of the subject in the practice of hypnosis to look at things objectively.

To make you realize you do not want to tremble at the sight of your phobias unnecessarily, and you do not want to indulge in something that jeopardizes your health.

FADING MEMORIES

The concept of false memory suggests that the human mind is not as sharp and accurate as you think. It tends to forget things. Also, over time perhaps it replaces things with something that didn't even happen, something comfortable to remember.

Also, it is used as a coping mechanism to fight trauma and let go of painful moments in life. Repressing the memories and getting on with life. However, it is a matter of dispute if ever, memory is entirely repressed.

So, for good or bad, our mind may replace memory with a false memory, and we may take it for our reality without realizing it. Hypnosis can help us make our way through this maze of memories and dissect for ourselves what is real and what is worth it.

One of the key aspects of hypnosis is working at the very core of our mind to unearth the foundation of any issues and any problem. And, when are working so closely to the mind, it becomes important to understand how this delicate and superiorly complex structure works.

Yes, the mind is reprogrammable. It can work out all the bias and heuristics and marshal your brain to effective use using hypnosis. This possibility opens hypnosis to several therapeutic uses. The one we have been inclined to discuss here is relevant to the weight loss application.

10

Conclusion

Thank you for reading this book. As you can see from these mindset exercises, a huge part of the weight loss process is going to be mental. You have to allow your mind to be open and let new thoughts come in so that you can reshape the way that you think. For so long, you might have been trapped in mental cycles that keep you in an unhealthy place, unable to keep the weight off.

No longer do you have to endure this kind of physical struggle. You are an incredibly powerful person. You can get everything that you want from this life with a healthy body that you create.

Make it a reality on your mind the fact that the journey to a healthy life and weight loss is long and has many challenges. Pieces of stuff we consider more important in life require our full cooperation towards them. Just because you are facing problems in your weight loss journey, it does not mean that you should stop, instead show and prove to the whole world how good your ability to handle constant challenges is—train your brain to know that eating healthy food together with functional exercises can work miracles.

Make it your choice and not something you are forced to do by a third party. Always tell yourself that weight loss is a long process and not an event.

Take every moment of your days to celebrate your achievements because these achievements are what piles up to massive victory. Make a list of stuff you would like to change when you get healthy; they may be small size clothes, being able to accumulate enough energy, participating in your most loved sports you have been admiring for a long period, or just feeling self-assured. Make these tips your number one source of empowerment; you will end up completing your 30 days without even noticing.

The problem is not the method or even the plan you are using to achieve it. The problem is in your mind. If you want to lose real body fat, reduce weight, create your ideal shape, and maintain your new look, it is essential to change your attitude towards food and exercise and your behavior towards both.

The best hypnosis programs for weight loss may require you to understand and replicate those mental processes used by people who have lost weight already. It might be tough leaving your comfort zone, but hypnosis will help you to reprogram your mind and install new thoughts that will become automatic habits once you identify the right behavior perfect for achieving your goal.

Eating less and adequately or exercising following a schedule won't be a dream anymore: hypnosis enhances and strengthens your will.

So, if you are worried about being overweight now, there is nothing wrong with undergoing hypnosis. After all, you have nothing to lose but weight.

Remember, you are not working on temporary changes but long-term goals. Therefore, lifestyle changes should not be stopped when the weight is lost. Always remind yourself of essential habits that are easier to follow daily. They include trusting yourself and the process by acknowledging that the real change lies in your hands. Stop complacency, get up, walk around for at least thirty minutes a day.

It's time that we use our minds to their full potential. Consistently take note of your thoughts and point out anytime that you might be having negative feelings passing through your brain. Look deep at the root to resolve these issues. The key to positive thinking is consistency.

It's not always about ignoring the bad and living in a way that you have a more delusional mindset. Positive outlooks can be very valid. Although there might be something negative happening in the world, being positive about it isn't the worst thing possible.

Ensure that you are always checking in with your emotions and staying true to yourself. Some days will be harder than others, so it's okay to just take a break to shut out the rest of the world for a moment.

What matters most at the end of the day is that you are making sure you are taking care of yourself first.

Your mind is the control center, and if this isn't properly managed, it will have dire effects on the rest of your body. Changing thoughts means changing habits, so give yourself some time in this transition period. You will be able to discover the healthy mentality needed to live a better life!

CPSIA information can be obtained
at www.ICGtesting.com
Printed in the USA
BVHW091101220221
600778BV00007B/592